A PLUM

MEN IN BED

BARBARA KEESLING, PH.D., is a well-known sexologist, therapist, writer, and educator with more than two decades of experience in the area of sexual health. She is the author of several bestselling books, including *How to Make Love All Night* and *The Good Girl's Guide to Bad Girl Sex.*

Praise for Barbara Keesling

"The best sex book I've read in years . . . a must-buy."
—Tracey Cox, author of *Hot Sex*,
on *The Good Girl's Guide to Bad Girl Sex*

"Dr. Keesling shows women how to prolong that exquisite state of excitement as long as possible before surrendering to the ultimate joys of intimate connection."
—John Gray, author of *Why Mars and Venus Collide*,
on *All Night Long*

"Grounded in solid psychological and physical research . . . an impressive reference and a source of support and encouragement."
—*Kirkus Reviews* on *Sexual Healing*

men in bed

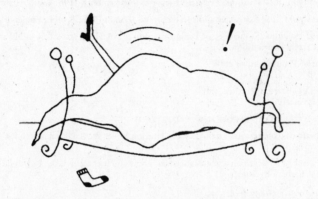

What Every Woman Needs to Know About Her Guy's Sexual Behavior

Barbara Keesling, Ph.D.

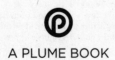

A PLUME BOOK

PLUME
Published by the Penguin Group
Penguin Group (USA) Inc., 375 Hudson Street, New York, New York 10014, U.S.A. •
Penguin Group (Canada), 90 Eglinton Avenue East, Suite 700, Toronto, Ontario, Canada
M4P 2Y3 (a division of Pearson Penguin Canada Inc.) • Penguin Books Ltd., 80 Strand,
London WC2R 0RL, England • Penguin Ireland, 25 St. Stephen's Green, Dublin 2,
Ireland (a division of Penguin Books Ltd.) • Penguin Group (Australia), 250 Camberwell
Road, Camberwell, Victoria 3124, Australia (a division of Pearson Australia Group Pty.
Ltd.) • Penguin Books India Pvt. Ltd., 11 Community Centre, Panchsheel Park, New
Delhi – 110 017, India • Penguin Group (NZ), 67 Apollo Drive, Rosedale, North Shore
0632, New Zealand (a division of Pearson New Zealand Ltd.) • Penguin Books (South
Africa) (Pty.) Ltd., 24 Sturdee Avenue, Rosebank, Johannesburg 2196, South Africa

Penguin Books Ltd., Registered Offices: 80 Strand, London WC2R 0RL, England

Published by Plume, a member of Penguin Group (USA) Inc. Previously published in a
Hudson Street Press edition.

First Plume Printing, April 2009
10 9 8 7 6 5 4 3 2 1

 REGISTERED TRADEMARK—MARCA REGISTRADA

The Library of Congress has catalogued the Hudson Street Press edition as follows:

Keesling, Barbara.
Men in bed : everything a woman needs to know about the good, the bad, and the
kinky / Barbara Keesling.
p. cm.
ISBN 978-1-59463-044-6 (hc.)
ISBN 978-0-452-29020-4 (pbk.)
1. Men—Sexual behavior. 2. Man-woman relationships. 3. Sex instruction for
women. I. Title.
HQ28.K44 2008
613.9'52—dc22   2008002655

Printed in the United States of America
Original hardcover design by Leonard Telesca

PUBLISHER'S NOTE
Every effort has been made to ensure that the information contained in this book is complete
and accurate. However, neither the publisher nor the author is engaged in rendering professional advice or services to the individual reader. The ideas, procedures, and suggestions
contained in this book are not intended as a substitute for consulting with your physician.
All matters regarding your health require medical supervision. Neither the author nor the
publisher shall be liable or responsible for any loss or damage allegedly arising from any information or suggestion in this book.

All names and identifying characteristics have been changed to protect the privacy of the
individuals involved.

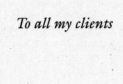

To all my clients

Contents

Acknowledgments

It takes a team to create a book. I would like to thank: my agent, Barbara Lowenstein, and the staff in her office for their professionalism, efficiency, and support; my editor, Cherise Davis, and everyone at Hudson Street Press who worked on the book; John Webb, for the many times he showed me how to work his fax when mine wouldn't do the job; Julia Sokol for her editorial skills and insight. Finally I would like to thank all the men and women who shared their ideas and talked to me about their sexual issues.

Reminder

We are living in the twenty-first century. This means that sexually transmitted diseases are a fact of life. I would like to remind everyone about condom use. I realize that with some of the techniques and exercises in this book, it is not always possible to use a condom. These are best done within the context of a committed sexual relationship in which both partners have had honest conversations about their exposure to STDs such as herpes and HPV and have had blood tests with negative results for the more serious STDs such as HIV.

Introduction

You are a lucky woman! Unlike women who lived in other eras, you have sexual choices. You can have sex with as many or as few men as you want. Unlike your grandmother, you were not led to believe that you would have to marry the first man who managed to undo the hooks on your bra. You are free to embrace and enjoy your sexuality. This is a great thing!

Nonetheless, we need to be realistic. The typical sexually active woman knows that the sex that is happening in her life doesn't always resemble the sex that is taking place in movies or current chick lit. Sleep with more than a few men, and the odds are that you are going to find yourself in a passionate embrace with a man who is "too quick." Go to bed with a few more, and you will probably meet a man who sometimes can't "get it up." You may even find yourself in a sexual relationship with someone who has a difficult time "getting it down." The more years you spend as a single, sexually active woman, the greater the likelihood of meeting a man who rarely (or never) wants sex as well as a man who always wants sex—sometimes the kinkier the better. Right now, in fact, you may even be in a relationship with one of these men. Even if you opt for one monogamous sexual relationship for the rest of your life, and have no intention of ever having sex with anyone else, you will find that the sexual attitude and behavior of the man in your bed change with time and age. You owe it to yourself to be prepared for all these possibilities.

At one time or another, most women will have to ask themselves whether they should try to forge successful, satisfying relationships with men who have sexual issues. As women, we tend to hold ourselves responsible for the sexual behavior of the men in our beds. We've been told things like "If your guy has limited desire, buy sexy lingerie, learn sensuous foot massage, purchase off-the-rack dominatrix outfits, and share your fantasies." This tends to reinforce a woman's belief that what happens in her bed is dependent on her ability to turn a man on. The opposite is also true. If the love of your life wants to have sex with everything that walks, you're told that you should take him to church or show him the way to a sexual addiction counselor or group. In all likelihood, at one time or another, every woman will ask herself, "Is it my fault?" or "What should I be doing differently?"

Complain to a friend that you are interested in a man who may not be the lover you dreamed of, and you may be advised to move on and look for greener pastures. The problem with that advice is that these problematic sexual partners may be men you like (and sometimes even love), real people with real concerns, not jokes on Comedy Central or *Sex and the City* reruns. In short, what can you expect from your love life? Is there such a thing as a normal sexual experience? If your experiences are less fulfilling than you expected, what can you do about it?

I started having sex at what I considered to be a late age (eighteen). I was definitely ready and eager before then, but the truth is that I couldn't talk anybody into it. As soon as I started having sex, I knew right away that I loved it! I immediately began looking forward to a lifetime of pleasure. I was lucky. My first few lovers fulfilled my expectations; they were so wonderfully normal that I took it for granted that all men were going to be that way. I didn't realize at the time how lucky I was.

Then, when I was still in my early twenties, there came the year that changed my life: That's when I became romantically involved with a group of men who were more than a little deficient in the bed department. It all started with Kevin, whose interest in sex was nonexistent. On a scale of one to ten, Kevin was about a minus two. He was followed by Harry, who couldn't (or wouldn't) ejaculate, and Brian, who I thought of fondly as the incredible two hundred pound, nonmoving man; he had an erection, but he would just lay there and didn't seem to know what to do with it. Brian was followed by several men with erection problems and several men with such serious alcohol problems that they couldn't get an erection.

You get the picture. For a while there, every man I met seemed to have a sexual issue or some other kind of personal issue that affected his sex life. My sex life was not turning out to be the exciting frolic I had expected. "What's going on here?" I wondered. Trying to understand what was going on in my own bedroom, I had started to do some reading and research, hoping to figure out what to do with some of these men, or at least the ones I was still interested in. I wanted to know more about sex and since my primary interest was heterosexual, I wanted more information about men. That's when I read an article in a local paper about a sex clinic that was employing sexual surrogate partners to help people with sexual problems. At the time, I was working for the post office, delivering mail in a little truck and wondering what I was going to do with the rest of my life. When I read the article about sexual surrogate partners, I really did have an "Aha!" moment. I said to myself, "I could do that . . . I could become a sexual surrogate and get a job having sex with men with problems. What a way to make a living!"

You see, I already felt as though I was doing exactly that—having sex with men with problems—but I wasn't getting paid!

Since my "Aha!" moment, I have spent much of my adult life studying male sexuality. Not only is it a subject about which I know a great deal, it is also the subject that is nearest and dearest to my heart. When I began my career in sexuality (sex researcher, educator, and therapist) as a sexual surrogate partner, I was in school studying for an Associate of Arts degree. I went on to earn a B.A., with a major in psychology, an M.A. in experimental psychology, and a Ph.D. in health psychology. In the past twenty years, I have taught all levels—graduate and undergraduate—of psychology and human sexuality. During my years as a sexual surrogate partner, I was associated with a sex therapy clinic where I was trained in a system based on the work of Masters and Johnson, pioneers in the behavioral treatment of sex problems. At this clinic I worked with hundreds and hundreds of men, women, and couples with all types of sexual concerns and issues. For many years I also had a private practice as a sex therapist. In addition to working with clients, in my personal life as a sexually active woman, I have been involved with many men who exhibited all types of sexual issues. In short, I have been to bed with great lovers, good lovers, bad lovers, boring lovers, clueless lovers, and everything in between.

In writing *Men in Bed*, it is my hope that I will help women be prepared for the men they will meet and the sex they will have. As far as sexuality is concerned, I have heard it all and seen it all. I want to share what I know.

men in bed

1

The Man in Your Bed:
Some Essential Information

Whether you are eighteen or eighty, each of the men you invite into your bed will play an essential role in how you think of yourself as a woman and sexual being. Some of these men will thrill you; some will enthrall you; some will confuse you; some will bore you; and some will probably repel you. Some will make you gasp with pleasure; others may make you consider abstinence as a life choice. Some will bring you joy; others will bring you pain. Your sexual partners influence more than your momentary pleasure; they have a profound effect on your self-esteem and sense of well-being.

Nobody could ever accuse me of being a prude. I've enjoyed a great deal of sex with many different men, but I've never underestimated the significance of any sexual encounter. Every time you have sex, it has the potential to change the rest of your life. You could fall in love; you could get pregnant; you could catch a disease; or you could become swept up in a heady combination of hormones, pheromones, and romantic fantasies so intense that you make a decision that alters the course of your life. Every woman needs to learn to be more practical and realistic about what happens in her bed. Sex is one of the most important things we do. It's never a casual act, even when it's with a complete stranger or someone you may never want to see again. If we are going to make informed decisions, we owe it to ourselves to learn as much as we can about male sexuality in general as well as the particular sexual patterns of the men with whom we are each sharing our individual beds.

Knowing more about male sexual behavior is a necessary ingredient in building good and satisfying relationships. I really love my car, for example. I love the way it looks, and I love the way it drives, but when the engine makes funny noises or the air conditioning breaks down, I take it to the mechanic who looks under the hood, tells me what's wrong, and fixes the problem—usually in the very same day. In order to have fun in my car, I don't need to know much more than that. I can't apply that same logic to the men in my life. I wish I could, but that's not how things work. When it comes to men, sex, and what's going on in the bedroom, I know there is no reliable "fix-it" service center and that women are pretty much on their own. Having some understanding of men—how they think and how they work—is an essential part of being able to have a good time in bed. The more information you have about male sexuality, the more secure, confident, and empowered you will be.

HIS SEXUAL ANATOMY: WHAT YOU NEED TO KNOW

One of the most obvious and important features of the male genitals is that they are immediately visible. When a guy takes his clothes off and looks down, he can see his penis. If he strolls around the apartment or a locker room, so can everyone else, particularly if he has a spontaneous erection that he can't hide or control. A little baby boy will frequently start touching and playing with his penis around the same time he starts reaching for a rattle or a teething biscuit. As soon as he is ready for potty training, his dad or another male will usually show him how to hold his penis and aim for the toilet bowl. All I'm saying by this is that men, unlike most women, are typically very familiar with how their genitals look and feel.

When you look at a man's nonerect penis, what you see is an external organ that on average measures a little less than four inches in length. Some men appear smaller; some appear larger. I should note here that when you look at a flaccid penis, you can't really tell how large it will become when aroused because typically a smaller nonerect penis will have a greater percentage increase as it becomes erect. External factors such as temperature can also cause a flaccid penis to appear smaller. Remember the *Seinfeld* episode in which Jerry's weekend date gets a glimpse of George Costanza's naked body after he emerges from a swim in cold water? She glances down at his genitals and her face registers disdain. Later George reminds everyone of the phenomenon known, as he puts it, as "shrinkage."

In the center of the penis, on the underside, is a tube called the urethra. This is the tube that carries urine and semen to the tip of the penis where they can exit via the urinary opening. Inside the penis itself are three separate cylinders of erectile tissue. The erectile tissue in all three of these cylinders contains small blood vessels. When a man becomes excited, the arteries leading to the penis widen, and blood flows into the cylinders. That's what causes his erection.

The penis, which is filled with nerves endings, is sensitive to both temperature and physical touch. This sensitivity is particularly true of the head of the penis. If a man has not been circumcised, there is also a loose, soft fold of protective skin (a foreskin) that covers the head of the penis.

The scrotum is a loose sac of skin that hangs directly underneath the penis; it contains the two male testes. Sperm and male hormones, particularly testosterone, are produced in the testes. By the way, just about every man you meet will refer to his testes pridefully as "my balls," or sometimes even "my boys." Like the penis, the scrotum itself is also sensitive to heat and cold. During the summer, for example, heat makes the scrotum relax and a man's testicles tend to hang rather loosely. When it is cold, the skin of the scrotum contracts and the testicles appear to be held tighter and closer to the body. Yet another example of George Costanza's "shrinkage." Exercise and arousal also cause the scrotum to contract. During sex, the skin of the scrotum contracts while increased blood flow causes the testes to enlarge. If you put your hand on your partner's scrotum before he ejaculates, you may notice that it feels as though it is scrunching up.

Many men derive sexual satisfaction when their partners touch the scrotum and gently squeeze their testes during sex. Some men may even like it when you pull or tug on the scrotum because it stimulates the testicles. There are other men, however, whose testicles are so sensitive to touch that they find this activity painful.

While we are talking about the sexual anatomy of men, I should mention the prostate gland, which also contributes to the male sexual response. It surrounds the urethra and is found below the bladder. The prostate gland is slightly larger than a walnut and produces an alkaline substance that, along with semen, is part of the seminal fluid a man ejaculates. When talking about seminal fluid, I should also mention the Cowper's glands; these produce a small amount of slippery pre-ejaculation fluid during sexual arousal. This fluid sometimes contains small amounts of sperm. Women need to know about this because this sperm can, of course, impregnate a woman before there is an ejaculation. This is one of the reasons why the withdrawal method of birth control sometimes fails.

You will very rarely hear younger men talking about their prostate glands. With age, however, the prostate can enlarge and become a health concern. Older men, for example, may begin to complain that an enlarged prostate is interfering with urination. All men need to check with their doctors to find out when they should start scheduling regular exams to screen for potential problems such as prostate cancer. Other conditions that can affect the male prostate include various forms of prostatitis, which is an inflammation of the prostate gland that can happen at any age.

HE HAS A POWERFUL SEXUAL MUSCLE—AND SO DO YOU

The pubococcygeal muscle, which I like to refer to familiarly as the PC muscle, is the sex therapist's secret weapon. Sometimes called the "pelvic floor" muscle, the PC muscle reaches from the pubic bone to the coccyx or tailbone, and it has sexual significance for *both* men and women. In men, the PC muscle is at the base of the penis; in women, it surrounds the vagina. It is the muscle you squeeze when you are trying to hold back urine. The muscle also contracts during orgasm. Women who have problems either with having orgasms or bladder control are often encouraged to start doing what are known as Kegel exercises. A strong, well-exercised PC muscle will improve orgasms and sex for both men and women.

If a man contracts or tenses his PC muscle, he can't get an erection. In fact, this is one of the ways in which erection enhancement drugs work; Viagra and other similar medications help relax the PC muscle so that blood can flow into the penis and cause it to become hard. When a man tenses his PC muscle during sex, it helps him hold back ejaculation. When a man is having an orgasm and ejaculating, the PC muscle spasms; this causes semen to be expelled from the penis. If a man has a great deal of control during sex and is able to last a long time, it is usually because he has taken the time to exercise his PC muscle and learned how to use his PC muscle to put off his ejaculation.

HE IS VERY AWARE OF HIS SEMEN

The first thing you need to know about semen is that the average guy takes his very seriously. Adolescent boys have even been known to have "circle jerks" in which they stand around in a group masturbating. Sometimes they compete as to who has the most semen or whose semen travels the longest distance. I know this seems gross to some women, but it's another example of the old saying "boys will be boys." Even if they never discuss this, men tend to pride themselves on the quantity and quality of their semen. I've heard men voice concerns such as "My semen isn't as thick this week as it usually is. I wonder what's wrong?" or "I don't think I have as much semen as other guys. Is there something I should take for that?"

The other thing you need to know about semen is that it's not all sperm. Seminal fluid is part sperm, which is produced in the testes, and part seminal plasma, which comes from a variety of sources including the prostate and the seminal vesicles. Semen is usually white in color, but it can also be grayish or yellowish. The taste, texture, smell, and thickness of a man's semen can be influenced by a variety of factors ranging from what he ate for dinner to how much alcohol he drank, or how long it's been since he last ejaculated.

There are some women who are allergic to the proteins found in semen. These women report pain, swelling, redness, and burning sensations. The symptoms will typically appear about half an hour after sex. In some instances, women are allergic to the semen of some men and not others. I've even heard women complain that they are only sensitive to a specific man's semen, and only under certain conditions.

TESTOSTERONE IS TO MEN WHAT ESTROGEN IS TO WOMEN

Testosterone, which is produced in a man's testicles, is the primary male hormone; men have ten to thirty times more testosterone than women. It is responsible for most of the qualities we associate with maleness, such as a deep voice and muscles. We've all heard about those athletes who take anabolic steroids—banned performance-enhancing drugs—in order to go faster, improve endurance, and build more muscle mass. Synthetic testosterone is an essential ingredient of these drugs.

Celebrated as the hormone that creates high levels of male desire and sexual enthusiasm, testosterone is also often associated with aggression and violence. In short, while you can thank testosterone for his bulging biceps and sexy baritone as well as his high energy and libido, many researchers also make a connection between testosterone and antisocial behavior.

In women, testosterone is produced in the ovaries; it also plays an important role in female sexuality. In fact, testosterone is sometimes prescribed for post-menopausal women who complain of a reduced libido. Women who take testosterone frequently report that it makes them more aggressive and competitive as well as more overtly sexual. Some of these women say that when they take the hormone, all they can think about is sex, and it gives them a better sense of what it feels like to have the sex drive of a man.

Somewhere between the ages of ten and sixteen, adolescent boys begin to experience the surges in testosterone that signal that they are on their way to becoming men. Everything is changing—not only their bodies, but the way they view the world. Testosterone stimulates the larynx, and their voices start to deepen; they begin to grow facial hair as well as body hair; and they notice that their genitals are developing. Some boys mature early; some mature later. For some males, sexual maturation is gradual and can take as long as five or six years, while others go through the entire process in a very short period of time. I remember the thirteen-year-old son of a friend of mine. His mother said that when she sent him off to summer camp, his pockets were filled with bubble gum and all he could think about was searching for frogs in the camp pond. When he returned eight weeks later, his pockets were filled with condoms (which a friend had told him he should always carry—just in case); he suddenly had an interest in television shows that featured girls with cleavage, and a well-read copy of *Playboy* was hidden in his duffel bag.

Think back to the kid in sixth or seventh grade who was a full head taller than anybody else and who was already starting to leer suggestively at the teacher. Surging testosterone explains his condition and his point of view. In the same class, remember the kid who was a foot shorter than his peers—the one who had no interest in competitive sports and even less interest in girls. His body had yet to start producing large amounts of testosterone.

Male testosterone production peaks in the twenties and begins to decline as a man ages, but it never disappears entirely. If a man visits a physician complaining about low sexual desire, it is customary for the doctor to test his testosterone levels to see if they are clinically low.

Here's the thing: You know how you have no control over whether you have big breasts, small breasts, or sagging breasts? That's just how much control men have over the amount of testosterone their bodies naturally produce. Men who produce large amounts of testosterone are more likely to be more interested in having sex more often and vice versa. It's a simple as that.

IT'S A RARE MAN WHO DOESN'T MASTURBATE

Most men start masturbating when they are in their early teens; it's an activity they continue for the rest of their lives. It's normal—men have always done it, and they will always do it. Back in the 1940s, the Kinsey Report showed that well over 95 percent of men masturbated; the more recent National Health and Social Life Survey in the 1990s confirmed that some things never change. A woman needs to know this so she doesn't get upset if she finds strange stains on the sheets, walks in on him in the shower, or wakes up in the middle of the night because her significant other's masturbation technique is making the mattress vibrate. Yes, it's normal for a man to masturbate even when he is in a sexual relationship. I've known so many women who have been hurt or insulted when they discovered how often their partners masturbate. A typical response: "Why does he have to masturbate? He has me!"

Men masturbate for a variety of reasons: Many men (as well as women), for example, say that the most intense orgasms they experience are with masturbation. Another reason for masturbating is the ease with which it can be accomplished. A guy can run through the shower in the morning and masturbate out of habit, with the same kind of regularity with which he brushes his teeth. Adolescents, for example, sometimes masturbate many, many times each day. Many of us remember Philip Roth's famous novel *Portnoy's Complaint*, which gives great emphasis to the amount of time his hero spends masturbating. In a chapter called "Whacking Off," Roth writes:

Then came adolescence—half my waking life spent locked behind the bathroom door, firing my wad down the toilet bowl, or into the soiled clothes in the laundry hamper, or *splat*, up against the medicine chest mirror, before which I stood in my dropped drawers so I could see how it looked coming out.

As men get older, they tend to masturbate less, but it's not at all unusual for some guys in their twenties or early thirties to masturbate once a day *and* also have sex with a partner one or more times a day. In short, frequency of masturbation can range from not at all to several times a day. This range is normal. A guy gets into trouble if his masturbation patterns become compulsive and/or if he is doing it mainly to relieve anxiety as opposed to having sexual pleasure.

Masturbation becomes an even more serious issue when a man always prefers masturbation, even if he has a willing partner. This indicates a sexual orientation called autoeroticism. I would advise any woman not to get involved with a man who has an autoerotic orientation. But just because you find out, in Roth's terminology, that your man is "whacking off" a little more often than you thought, this is no cause for concern.

When I was working as a sexual surrogate partner, I would start all my clients with at least one session devoted to masturbation. I would tell them just to pretend that I wasn't there and to do what they would do if they were all alone. I must have watched hundreds of men masturbating. By watching a guy masturbate, I could tell a great deal about how he approached sex with a woman. I could also see if he had any patterns that were getting in the way of his sexual pleasure. What I saw truly surprised me. I was amazed, for example, by how quickly many men masturbated. Some went from arousal to ejaculation in a matter of a couple of minutes or less. I was also taken aback by how roughly some men handle their genitals; there seems to be a belief that faster and harder is the way to go. When a man manhandles his penis in this way, he may ultimately have a more difficult time having good sex with a woman because he expects intercourse to duplicate that level of physical stimulation, and it doesn't.

I discovered that most men masturbate by putting one hand around the shaft of the penis and moving it up and down. This is by far the most common style. Some men concurrently stroke the head of the penis, fondle the scrotum, or use a finger to stimulate the anus. Some men will stroke themselves while sitting up or standing, but most prefer to lie on their backs. Many men regularly masturbate in the bathtub or shower because it's easy to clean up. Some men clean up afterward using a sock. Some men even masturbate into a sock. I'm not kidding. I guess they figure they were going to throw it in the laundry anyway. Some men masturbate with two hands, rubbing the penis as though they were rubbing two sticks together trying to start a fire. (Maybe they started their masturbation habits at Boy Scout camp?)

Men frequently use pornography and/or fantasy as an adjunct to masturbation. I'm sure there are some men who use inflatable dolls or artificial vaginas, but they haven't crossed my path. Most men use some kind of lubrication. If they run out of their preferred brand, they will generally just use saliva or improvise with something out of the kitchen, like vegetable oil.

In all my years as a sex therapist and surrogate partner, I've had only one client who masturbated in a way that I considered weird. He would lie on his stomach and rub his penis against the bed. There is nothing wrong with this, but this man also had a great many sexual anxieties and fears, and he had been masturbating in this fashion for so long that he wasn't able to make the transition to having sex with a woman. Everything he did, from the amount of pressure he put on his penis to the speed with which he masturbated, exacerbated his problem. I always advised clients that the most effective way for a man to masturbate is to mimic intercourse as best he can with a lot of lubrication and stopping and starting in order to prolong the sensation.

MOST MEN HAVE SEXUAL FANTASIES

Many men always rely on fantasies to bring them to orgasm; others never do. Some men only use these fantasies when they are masturbating; others focus on their favorite fantasies even when they are having sex. Some men find a fantasy that works for them when they are still teenagers, and they cling to it forever after. It could be something as simple as a *Playboy* photograph or a simple fantasy such as having intercourse with the sexy French teacher they remember from sophomore year or spending a night in the local motel with their best friend's older sister. It worked for them when they were fifteen, and it still works at fifty. Other men vary their fantasies throughout the years and choose from a wide assortment. There are a fair number of men, for example, who change their fantasies daily, routinely imagining themselves having sex with just about every woman they meet—and in every conceivable position. I have found that men are much more likely than women to fantasize about sex with unknown partners. Sometimes they don't even need to put a face on these random female images. Other than that, male fantasies are similar to female fantasies—forbidden sex, forbidden partners, or sex with someone you love. Men frequently fantasize about being physically and emotionally dominant.

Men have told me some peculiar fantasies over the years. I always remember the guy who told me that he couldn't have an orgasm unless he fantasized about beating his penis against a clipboard. (Maybe he eventually hooked up with someone who worked for a market research company?) I also remember a client who dreamed about having a woman perform oral sex on him while he did chin-ups on a bar. In a perfect world, he would have connected with a personal trainer.

THE STAGES OF AN ERECTION

Most women don't think too much about how or why a man gets an erection, but I think knowing more about how men function helps women become better and more confident lovers. I describe the process of male erection as having four stages.

Stage One: Initiation. This is the stage at which a man receives some form of sexual stimulation. He sees, hears, touches, or thinks about something that excites him, and his penis begins to react.

Stage Two: Filling. Blood starts to flow into the penis, which begins to harden accordingly. On a scale numbered 1–10, number 1 would be no erection; 2–4 would indicate that blood is beginning to flow into the penis and it is becoming firmer.

Stage Three: Rigidity. Once blood flow to the penis is established, valves at the base of the penis close off to keep the blood in the penis. Use that same 1–10 scale. 5 would describe a penis that is hard enough to begin to proceed with sex. 6–10 would describe a penis that is definitely hard enough for intercourse. A penis that is at 10 is so erect that if you were to push down on it, it would spring back. Some erections are so firm that they may not move at all.

WHY DOES A PENIS BECOME ERECT?

A penis becomes erect because of physical or mental stimulation. Sometimes erections occur because the penis itself is being touched or stroked and this causes a spontaneous physical reflexive response. Other times, erections occur as a result of mental stimulation because the man is having a fantasy or thinking about sex. Most often, erections happen because there is a combination of physical and mental stimulation. Young men frequently become erect with only the slightest stimulation of any kind, whether it be mental or physical. I was recently amused while watching an episode of the HBO series *Big Love*; in it, the adolescent son struggles with a penis that responds too quickly. In woodshop one day, the instructor is using a drill to cut through a piece of wood. The sight of the drill going in and out of the wood is enough to cause the boy's penis to become erect. Embarrassed, he finishes the class clutching his books down below his belt.

A man once told me that when he was fourteen, all he had to do was glance at a woman's breasts and he would have an erection. He said that during school, he would always keep his eyes down, looking at his desk or even the floor for fear of becoming accidentally aroused and consequently embarrassed. People thought he was a real jerk who wouldn't make eye contact. Typically, as men become older they require more stimulation, whether it is mental or physical. A young man, for example, might become erect from the feel of a soft fabric on his penis or from the sight of a young woman walking down the school hallway. An older man might require oral stimulation or intercourse combined with a highly charged fantasy or pornography.

During the most heated session of lovemaking, it is not uncommon for a man's penis to go through varying degrees of hardness and softness. When you are performing oral sex on him, for example, he may be rock hard, but if you stop doing that while he concentrates on your pleasure, he may lose part of his erection. That doesn't mean that he is losing interest in the sex. It simply means that his penis is not receiving the same kind of physical stimulation, so his arousal level is slightly diminished.

UNDERSTANDING LEVELS OF AROUSAL

In order to help you develop greater awareness of levels of arousal, I suggest thinking of arousal on a scale from 1 to 10, with 1 indicating no arousal and 10 being orgasm. I have written this emphasizing the male response, but it works for women too.

Level 1: No arousal.

Levels 2–3: Low level of arousal. The arousal level is still low and intermittent enough so that he can pretty easily change direction and start focusing on food or television or anything else instead of sex.

Levels 4–5: Arousal has now become a constant, but it's still at a low level.

Levels 6–7: Arousal is steady and moderate, and he doesn't want the stimulation to stop.

Level 8: He is aware of a quickened heartbeat; if he talks, he may sound as though he is out of breath.

Level 9: He is very close to orgasm. Anything beyond this point and orgasm is inevitable.

Level 10: Bingo!

THERE IS A DIFFERENCE BETWEEN ORGASM AND EJACULATION

Honest. I'm not kidding you. Ejaculation is a localized genital response. It happens when the PC muscle spasms and sends semen out of the penis. Orgasm is a full body response that includes rapid heart rate, intense pleasure, and a physical sense of release. Most of the time, the experience of orgasm and ejaculation happen closely together so even men are not always aware that they are two distinct events. In the course of a lifetime, however, most men will have the experience of ejaculating without feeling all those wonderful sensations that accompany orgasm. I should also add that there are some men (probably between 5 to 10 percent) who are able to have one or more orgasms without ejaculating. These men have usually trained themselves to do this. It's called male multiple orgasm or nonejaculatory orgasm.

EVERY MAN HAS A REFRACTORY PERIOD

If you've had an orgasm at ten o'clock in the morning, how long will it be before you are able to have another one? Are you ready for another one in minutes? Hours? Days? The male refractory period is the amount of time after a man has ejaculated before he is able to get aroused again. Women, of course, can usually have sex immediately even if they are not able to climax. Men have a different physiology and may be incapable of managing another erection for hours or even days. Some women say that the clitoris is so incredibly sensitive right after sex that even being touched can border on painful. Some men describe the same sensations when talking about the penis.

The male refractory period varies greatly from man to man and is dependent on a wide variety of factors including age, testosterone levels, general health, and psychological attitude. A very young man, for example, may be able to have an erection, achieve orgasm, and be ready to go again in minutes. Some young men can have sex many times in a twenty-four-hour period, reaching orgasm each time. I've certainly known men who were capable of five or six orgasms during a twenty-four-hour time frame. But as these men age, their patterns may change. The guy who was capable of making love four times a night when he was twenty-five may only be capable of doing it twice at thirty-eight. Another typical pattern is reflected by the man who has sex once with an orgasm at, let's say, ten P.M. He may have another erection at eleven P.M. and make love for an hour without being able to have an orgasm; he may need to wait until morning before having sex with an ejaculation. Then he may feel that he needs another forty-eight hours before he is again interested in sex.

After having sex, a fifty-year-old man may need to wait at least twenty-four to forty-eight hours before he is able to get an erection and ejaculate. The seventy-year-old man may be happier waiting a week or even more.

YOUR GUY FROM TWENTY TO SEVENTY AND BEYOND—WHAT TO EXPECT

Although all men are different and have different levels of desire, testosterone, and sexual energy, there are a few generalities that we can make. Here is an overview of what you can expect sexually from the man in your bed as he ages.

Your guy from 20–29

Remember that testosterone peaks in the early to midtwenties, so this is when your guy is at his sexual prime in terms of his hormones, desire, and the ability to have frequent erections. In fact, he is often still able to have an erection just by thinking about sex. He is likely to experience premature ejaculation at least some of the time. If he has problems having an erection at this age, his issues are more likely to be psychological than physical. He may have already had several previous sexual partners (the twenty-something-year-old men in my class, for example, report having had an average of ten partners for sexual intercourse), but he may still be inexperienced in terms of how to please a woman. He will also have a different attitude toward sexuality than older men. He, for example, matured during a time when oral sex was more frequently identified with heavy petting than with actual sex. Men in this age group have the drill about using condoms for protection against STDs embedded in their brains, so they are more apt to always carry condoms. Depending on where he is in his twenties, he may not have yet had a serious girlfriend or been in a long-term relationship. My experience with this age group has shown that what they lack in experience, they more than make up for with enthusiasm, strong desire, and admirable energy. These guys also still tend to masturbate with regularity and frequently use porn.

Men in this age group sometimes use alcohol and recreational drugs, but unless a guy is "wasted," his sexuality will rarely be totally compromised. If he is taking Viagra, he is doing it for recreational purposes, not because he needs it. Research shows that sexual addictions and kinks are established very early (often in childhood), but in my experience, guys in their twenties still have so much natural sexual energy that they are less likely to depend on full-blown S&M or other forms of kinky behavior to get aroused.

I think it's important to note that the guy from twenty to twenty-nine is unlikely to have medical problems that interfere with his sex life. In fact, he probably can't even imagine the possibility of that happening.

Your guy from 30–39

As far as I'm concerned, thirty-five is the new twenty-one! The thirties are a fabulous decade for a man. He still has much of his youthful sex drive and the ability to have an erection. His ejaculatory urge may have declined somewhat since his twenties, and he is less likely to worry about ejaculating prematurely.

If he drinks too much or indulges in recreational drugs, he will probably notice that his erection is not as reliable as it once was. When the thirty-something-year-old man feels his sexual abilities are declining, he may rely more on porn or fantasies. If he has an underlying preoccupation with kinky sex or sexual exploration, this is the time when these interests will probably begin to come more to the forefront.

Many men in this age group feel ready to settle down (at least temporarily) with one person, and the average thirty-year-old is likely to be in a serious relationship or at least to have already had one. He is also probably a more experienced and confident lover. If he is a parent or wants to become one, sex may have developed more serious overtones; fatherhood will definitely make a difference in his sex life. His work may be taking up more of his day, and for the first time, he may sometimes be so tired that he occasionally complains about diminished desire. When he was twenty, perhaps he had an erection just by thinking about sex. Now, thinking about sex alone may not always be enough, and his penis may require some direct physical stimulation. Something to remember with some men in this age bracket and beyond, however, is that they may not have been made as aware of STDs as younger men, and don't always take condom use seriously.

Your guy from 40–49

Women tend to find men in their forties very exciting and sexually stimulating. Unfortunately, however, many men in this decade don't always feel that sexy. That's because this is when most men begin to notice that they are having fewer spontaneous erections and that their erections are not as frequent or as firm as they once were. If the man in your bed is in this age group, it may take him longer to have an orgasm and his ejaculation may have less volume. He definitely has lower testosterone, and he may start noticing that he doesn't have the high levels of enthusiasm and desire he once had. He may also have some physical issues caused by sports injuries. A trick knee or shoulder, for example, may cause him to avoid certain positions. Perhaps he even requires something like arthroscopic or knee replacement surgery. Crutches, canes, and needing somebody to lean on, even temporarily, can change his view of himself and his partner. He may start losing his hair or become aware of other physical changes. This is the time when some men experience the traditional midlife crisis. If this is the case, he may look for ways to prove himself sexually or show that he is still in the game.

If the forty-something-year-old guy drinks too much, the chances are really high that his erection will falter. If he is working too hard or is under too much stress, his erection will suffer. He will probably experience the first signs of waning sexual desire at times when he can't use fatigue as an excuse. Some men respond to this by hunkering down with their partners; others feel a need to do whatever they can to fan their sexual energy. Some guys become more involved with experimental or kinky sex; others may start noticing younger women.

This is also the age when a variety of physical ailments such as high blood pressure may become bigger issues. In terms of sex, the medications that are given for some of these ailments can affect all aspects of male sexuality—desire, erection, and ejaculation.

Your guy from 50–59

This can be a great age, and men in their fifties often evolve into astounding lovers. Although their erection abilities may have declined somewhat (not as often, not as hard, and requiring direct physical stimulation), when it comes to pleasing women, many men in this age group are strongly motivated. The fifty-something-year-old man is also fairly experienced and often knows exactly what to do and how to do it. Nonetheless, testosterone levels are definitely traveling in a downward direction and men in this age group frequently visit their doctors to see about sexual enhancement drugs.

The good news is that the fifty-something-year-old man has truly started to mellow; his testosterone levels will probably be reduced, and he may be less aggressive and more willing to cuddle and be affectionate without having sex. I should also mention that when it comes to sex, the fifty-year-old is less likely to treat his body as though it is a machine; if he is having any physical or emotional problems, it will have an impact on his sexuality. Having said this, I should also say that I have found that men in this age group are particularly willing to learn new techniques to please a woman.

Your guy at 60+

Twenty years ago if a sixty-year-old man had difficulties with his erections, he had few available options. Remember that the statistics say that 50 percent of all men over the age of forty will have some form of erectile dysfunction. This is a huge statistic, and many of these over-forty men are, indeed, in their sixties or older. Years ago, I remember meeting many men who were still very eager to enjoy sex, but couldn't get erections. Some of them seemed to spend huge amounts of their spare time researching penile implants. Viagra changed all that. This is good news! Men in this age bracket are frequently willing to learn new ways of pleasing a woman and they tend to have let go of many of their inhibitions. There are, however, physical issues that some of these guys will face. Many of these revolve around problems with the prostate. Fortunately, the erection-enhancing drugs have helped many men, including those who have received treatment for health problems related to the prostate, even serious ones like cancer.

MOST MEN HAVE SOME SEXUAL INSECURITIES

Since sexuality is such a crucial component of masculinity, males feel pressured to act interested in sex whether or not they really are. They have to join in the jokes and banter. "Getting any, Fred?" "Oh yeah, more than I know what to do with." And they have to face the derision of their peers if they're still—God forbid—virgins at the advanced age of eighteen or twenty-three. This is a great setup for faking, lying, and feeling inadequate.

—Bernie Zilbergeld

You know the ways in which you are sexually insecure. Perhaps you are uncomfortable taking your clothes off in a lighted room; perhaps you worry about the size of your breasts or your tummy sags; perhaps you are insecure about telling your lover how to bring you to orgasm; perhaps you don't know how to talk about sex; perhaps you worry that your vagina is too big or too small or too dry or too wet. Perhaps your mother convinced you that you always needed to hide your thighs; perhaps you have been intimidated by all those perfect bodies in women's magazines. No woman is so secure that she is completely without some kind of sexual concern or worry. Men are no different. In fact, they may be even more insecure.

In his book *The New Male Sexuality*, Bernie Zilbergeld quotes an article Bill Cosby wrote for *Playboy* some years ago. In it, Cosby talked about his embarrassment at being a young man, going over to his girlfriend's house to have sex, and not even knowing what sex was. He wrote:

So now, I'm walkin' and I'm trying to figure out how to do it. And when I get there, the most embarrassing thing is gonna be when I have to take my pants down. See, right away, then, I'm buck naked in front of this girl. Now, what happens then? Do you . . . do you just . . . I don't even know what to do. . . . I'm gonna just stand there and she's gonna say, You don't know how to do it. And I'm gonna say, Yes I do, but I forgot. I never thought of her showing me, because I'm a man and I don't want her to show me—I don't want nobody to show me, but I wish somebody would kinda slip me a note.

The thing is, men are expected to know what to do, even when they are clueless. Some men are fortunate; they partner up with women and they learn. Some men are so insecure about sex that it takes years before they reach the point where they don't need somebody to "slip them a note."

The most common male insecurity has to do with the size of his penis. Does it "measure up"? Women never quite understand this concern and tend to think it's a joke, but trust me, it's real. That's why most men like it when their partners compliment them for having an attractive penis. I'm not kidding about this either. Don't you like it when a man tells you that you have beautiful breasts? The same kind of psychology is working for men. I'm not saying that you should lie and tell a man that he has the biggest penis you've ever seen when it isn't true, but it doesn't hurt to say something complimentary about how it looks or how your partner uses it. Even if you're relatively inexperienced (or don't want to appear so experienced that you scare him), you can say something along the lines of, "I haven't seen that many penises, but yours seems really terrific!" Again, trust me, men like that kind of thing.

Insecurity about penis size is part and parcel of that larger insecurity known as performance anxiety, which most men carry with them. All it means is that the guy feels that somebody (his partner) is watching him and grading him on what he does in bed. Does he have the right moves? Is he spending enough time on foreplay? Is he able to get erect? Is he able to sustain an erection? Does he come too soon? Does he know what to do with his mouth and his body? Does he know how to bring a woman to orgasm? That's a lot of pressure for a man to carry, and just about every man is aware of it and develops coping mechanisms to deal with his fears and anxieties. At one end of the spectrum, he may, for example, cover up his anxieties with bravado and regularly make sexual advances to strange women; at the other end, he may be so shy about sex that he actually avoids contact. ·

A primary reason why so many men have sexual insecurities is that they rarely have conversations about sex and are not sure about what is considered "normal" behavior in bed. Talking about our sexual habits, especially insecurities, is the deepest or most intimate level of self-disclosure. This is no less true for men than it is for women. Men usually don't even talk honestly to each other, and when they do, what they say tends to be handled as a joke or with humor. They are frequently embarrassed about showing any insecurity or exposing what they don't know. In my experience, they tend to exaggerate their lifetime number of partners in order to look good. They actually calculate their lifetime number of intercourse partners differently than women do. Men tend to count a near miss as a hit, for example. Women, on the other hand, may do the exact opposite because society often wants women to appear less sophisticated in terms of sex.

Some men are nervous about having conversations about sex because they don't know what's acceptable to say. For many, viewing pornography is the only real exposure they have to discussions about sexuality. When it comes to talking about sex without a pornographic context, they aren't even sure which words to use and which might be offensive to some people. The typical male is also frequently reluctant to talk to a woman about his true sexual desires. Why? Because he's afraid she might think he's a pervert or what he says is totally gross. His logic goes like this: "If she thinks I'm obsessed with sex, she might not want to have sex with me."

There is another phenomenon that explains why men don't talk about sex. It's called pluralistic ignorance. Pluralistic ignorance describes a situation when you don't do something because you think other people aren't doing it, or, conversely, you do something because you think everybody else is doing it. The social stereotype is that "men don't talk about sex with women," only with other guys in a locker room fashion. So men don't talk because they think other men aren't doing it. Men also rarely discuss their sexual performance or behavior except in general terms. "I always have trouble the first time," or "I can never have that second ejaculation," or "Sometimes I have trouble ejaculating." There are exceptions, of course. I remember one guy (who I never had sex with, but everybody else I know did). He couldn't shut up about his sexual issues. He even did a performance piece in New York about it—on stage, naked. As one of my friends said, he was an expert on natural foods and unnatural acts. But he was the exception, and I never believed a word he said about anything anyway.

EVERY MAN HAS AN ATTITUDE TOWARD WOMEN AND SEX

By the time the average guy arrives in a high school locker room, he has developed an attitude toward his penis and sex that is, at least in part, dependent on his family's attitude toward the body and sex. Did his parents, for example, use baby talk to describe his penis—as in your "little peeny weeny"? Did his mother stop him every time he touched himself, or did his father walk around naked while scratching his own balls? Did his parents talk about sex? Did they make judgments on women who were openly sexual? Did his parents give him information about birth control and safe sex, or did they leave it up to him to figure these things out on his own? All of these things are going to have something to do with how he feels about women, his penis, and sex in general.

Most studies, for example, show that preferences for sexual behaviors—whether they be kinky or traditional—are established by early puberty. If a guy can, for example, only have an erection or orgasm in a sado-masochistic environment, this tendency has its origins in his own particular background and involves a combination of factors. For example, some early emotional trauma may have disrupted a normal developmental pattern. Or he may have been exposed to particularly exciting sexual stimulation at a young age and may have fixated on some element of this stimulation. Some scientists also argue that brain patterns are the operative factor in sexual behavior; some of us are hardwired for traditional sexual behavior while others are not.

When a woman is starting, or deciding whether to continue having, a sexual relationship with a man, one of the things she needs to consider is whether the guy's attitude or behavior makes her reasonably happy, or is so over-the-top that she doesn't want to go any further. No question about it, some sexual issues are cognitive-behavioral and can be worked out by two well-intentioned people who want to improve a sexual relationship and are willing to think and talk about what they are doing. Other issues, however, reveal deep-seated psychological problems that a woman might reasonably find scary. These are the kinds of problems that may require that the man enter long-term therapy.

Back in the 1970s, a sex therapist named Jack Annon came up with a system for determining what level of help a client needs. It's called the PLISSIT model. These initials stand for Permission, Limited Information, Specific Suggestions, and Intensive Therapy.

Permission: Some guys' issues are so minor that they don't need much more than verbal permission to change in order to do so. Simon, for example, has never performed oral sex on a woman because he isn't sure how to do it and he is too shy to initiate this activity on his own. However, once his partner talks about oral sex, and indicates that this is something she wants, Simon is relieved and happy both to discuss it and to do it. In fact, he is thrilled. This is a simple cognitive-behavioral problem.

Limited Information: Some guys have sexual issues because they are clueless and don't know how to find out what to do. A man, for example, may stop having sex because he is stressed at work and doesn't respond to sexual stimuli as quickly as he once did. He may be so surprised by having diminished desire that he becomes nervous about having sex for fear he won't have an erection. Sometimes, all this kind of man needs is some limited information about realistic expectations along with relaxation techniques and his behavior changes.

Specific Suggestions: For example, let's take a guy who thinks that his partner wants fifteen minutes of hard thrusting, when she really doesn't. He might have no difficulty altering the way he has intercourse if his partner tells him that she would be happier with a change in tempo and shows him how she wants to be touched.

Intensive Therapy: Some sexual issues are so huge that they can only be handled by therapy with appropriate professionals.

This book will focus on people who need either limited information or specific suggestions.

2

The Overexcited Man

Not that long ago, I talked with a group of women about what was going on in their bedrooms. I asked them this question: When you or your friends talk about the sexual behavior of your husbands, boyfriends, and lovers, what is your most common complaint? I wasn't surprised when they began talking about all the men they knew who were so excited that they had no control. "He could barely get it out of his pants!" was a common theme.

Take Debra, for example. She liked Sam almost from the moment they first made eye contact. It was the middle of July and both were at the beach alone; Debra was struggling to get her umbrella secured in the sand when Sam came over to help her. He seemed to be the kind of guy who liked helping people, and Debra really appreciated and respected that quality. After the umbrella was stable, Sam sat down on her blanket and they started talking. It turned out that they both lived in the same neighborhood and even had friends in common. Sam seemed funny and smart and cute. When Sam asked Debra if she would go out with him, she said yes without any hesitation. She thought it was her lucky day!

For their first date, they went to a party at Sam's cousin's house where everybody made Debra feel very welcome. Sam was definitely somebody Debra could think about long-term. When Sam kissed

Debra good night, she practically quivered. He called the next day and asked her out again, and again she said yes. For their second date, Deb asked him to come with her to see her brother's baseball team play. After the game, Debra introduced Sam to her brother, and they seemed to get along immediately. Once again, Sam kissed Debra good night—several times. Once again, Debra vibrated. He was a great kisser!

The other thing that Debra liked about Sam was that he seemed to like her as much as she liked him. They began e-mailing and talking on the phone from the day they met. For their third date, they planned to spend the afternoon at the same local beach and then go back to Sam's apartment and order a pizza for dinner. Debra expected that once they were behind closed doors together, things would get more sexually serious. She had several creative fantasies in her head about what might happen between the two of them. She imagined that they would kiss a lot, share a pizza, maybe drink some wine and end up making love.

Forget about the pizza! Sam started kissing Debra the minute they walked into his apartment. Debra was very responsive and very excited, but she had fantasized that their first sexual experience together would be slow and easy. Instead, Sam hurried her into the bedroom. All Debra had on was a bathing suit and a cover-up so she didn't have much clothing to remove. Neither did Sam. After a few passionate kisses and some disrobing, Debra could see that Sam had a very firm erection. She was glad that she didn't have to remind him to put on a condom, but within three seconds of his doing so, he fell on top of her on the bed. He inserted his penis and started moving. Debra didn't even have enough time to adjust her body. Sam moved back and forth a few times, shuddered and grimaced, and Debra realized that he had ejaculated.

"That was great!" Sam told her as he rolled over onto his back and jumped out of bed. "I'm starving! What do you want on your pizza?"

"Wow," Debra thought to herself as she watched Sam's cute butt disappear into the bathroom, "that was a little quick." She tried to force herself to start thinking about pizza as opposed to what was (or wasn't) going on between her legs. "That was just the first time," she told herself. "First times don't count. It's bound to get better."

Well, Debra has now gone out with Sam four more times, but each time they get together, the sex is almost exactly the same—very quick! Debra wishes that she had somebody she could really talk to about what is going on with Sam in bed, but she hesitates to discuss it even with her closest friends. She doesn't want her friends to start laughing; she likes Sam and she doesn't want to expose his issues to the world. Besides, if she were to end up with Sam long-term, she wouldn't want everybody to know that she and Sam were having bad sex. But she definitely needs more information. What is Sam's problem? Even more important, is there anything she can do about it?

PREMATURE EJACULATION—WHAT IS IT?

Premature ejaculation, also known as PE, affects a large percentage of all men. According to the latest studies I've seen, it's at 28 percent. That's more than one in four men. Read that again: one in four. It's the most common male sexual concern. If you have sex with more than a few men, the chances that you will find yourself in bed with a guy with PE are spectacularly good. There is nothing complicated about defining PE. When a man has PE, all it means is that he is quickly aroused and goes through the stages of arousal leading up to ejaculation so rapidly that he cannot sustain an erection long enough to satisfy his partner. Some men with PE are so sensitive to physical stimulation that they ejaculate within a few seconds of penetration. Others can last a little bit longer; still others go through the stages of arousal so rapidly that they regularly ejaculate before the penis even makes contact or gets inside a woman's vagina.

Why do men have PE?

When I first began working as a sexual surrogate partner, one of the things that surprised me most was the number of men who appeared to have PE. The other thing that surprised me was how normal and average these guys were. I guess I was still clinging to a dated view that said that sexual difficulties were primarily psychological and reflected deep-seated issues. I remember hearing myths like "Men with PE are afraid of women—or afraid of sex." I didn't find this to be true.

In my experience, most guys with PE got that way as a result of their earliest sexual experiences, conditioning, and habits that become ingrained. Think about what goes on with adolescent boys, who typically start masturbating in their early teens. They are often uncomfortable about doing it and even a little bit guilty. They certainly don't want to get caught in the act by other family members. Visualize Brother in the bathroom while Sister bangs on the door, yelling to their mother, "Ma, make him get out of there!" With that kind of experience, easily aroused adolescent males frequently learn to ejaculate as quickly as possible to lessen the risk of somebody barging in. In short, the average guy learns how to do it "quick." This common approach to masturbation doesn't help young males learn anything about slow arousal or maintaining an erection for longer periods of time.

Under the best of circumstances, young males tend to ejaculate with greater speed than would be desirable for a long, sensuous session of lovemaking. As they get older, through a process of trial and error, most males learn how to slow down their arousal, get some control over their erections, and sidestep around that point of no return—but some of them don't. Men with chronic, longstanding PE tend to be just normal guys who have never learned how to avoid the arousal point of no return. I liken this to a man trying to ride a sophisticated multi-speed racing bike without bothering to learn how to use the brakes or gear shifts.

Does anxiety play a role in PE?

While I don't believe that PE usually has deep-seated psychological roots, PE will definitely increase a man's general anxiety and emotional stress about sex. Much of this stress is situational and has little or nothing to do with an underlying "fear of women." Let's take Debra's boyfriend, Sam, for example. Sam has always been easily aroused, and he discovered this when he was a young teenager dating for the first time. Some of his friends would talk about the "boners" they had when they were necking and making out with girlfriends for extended periods of time. Sam knew that he couldn't afford to "make out" with his girlfriend on the couch in her family room. If he did so, he ran the risk of ejaculating all over himself, her, and the couch. Eventually, Sam got into the habit of masturbating right before he went out on dates. This helped a little, but never so much that he felt totally comfortable about risking too much body contact with a woman. Sam's concerns about his quick ejaculations were confirmed the first times he engaged in physical intimacy with a woman. His first experience with oral sex, when he was still a teenager, was pretty much a disaster. He still remembers the way his girlfriend jerked her head back when he ejaculated seconds after she started. He could tell that she wasn't happy. In fact, she appeared to be grossed out.

As much as Sam currently wants to enjoy having a woman perform oral sex on him, he is so nervous about having his partner laugh at him or get turned off that he pretty much avoids oral sex. As far as intercourse is concerned, if Sam is going out on a date, he masturbates first. He always uses a condom because he has discovered this may buy him an extra few seconds. As you can imagine, all this worry about his ejaculation has affected him; as much as he wants and enjoys sex, just thinking about it is enough to make him tense.

A guy with PE has a variety of things to think about. He knows that he can't control the speed with which he ejaculates; he also knows that people joke about "premature ejaculators." He can tell time as well as his sexual partners can; he knows the difference between ten seconds and ten minutes. He knows that he has a difficult time satisfying most women the way they want to be satisfied. All of this is anxiety producing. Men with extreme cases of PE might tell you that they are often nervous or afraid to be around a woman, but this is not because they don't like women. They often say that it's because they like them so much that the slightest physical contact can make them aroused, and arousal is followed too quickly by ejaculation. And, yes, this makes sexual situations even more stressful.

One of the main problems with men with PE is that their experiences with sex have given them intense anxiety about being in the vagina and they are overwhelmed both psychologically and physically by what the vagina feels like. That's why I always encourage men with PE issues to try to have as much intercourse as possible. Even if they ejaculate rapidly, intercourse will help them become more comfortable with the sensation of being inside a vagina. This, in itself, is taking a big step forward in overcoming PE.

Are there some men whose PE makes them so anxious that they lose their erections? Absolutely. These men are then in an even more unpleasant situation. When they are with a woman, instead of trying to slow down, they may consciously start trying to speed up so that they don't lose their erection before having an orgasm or ejaculating.

Does PE go away as a man gets older?

This has a yes and no answer. There is no question about it, the length of time it takes for a man to become aroused increases as he ages. Having said that, I have successfully treated men in their sixties and seventies who spent a lifetime struggling with PE. In fact, PE can become more complicated for a man as he approaches his fifties or sixties because then he may also have difficulties getting and maintaining an erection.

Are there any medical conditions that cause PE?

I know of only two medical conditions that cause PE—alcohol withdrawal and opiate withdrawal. Alcohol and opiates both slow reflexes down. When you quit or try to withdraw from these addictions, it can speed up the ejaculatory reflex. These instances of PE are usually temporary.

HOW DO MEN HANDLE THEIR PROBLEMS WITH PE?

Men with PE rarely have anyone with whom they can discuss this issue. Certainly, it's not the kind of thing the average guy can comfortably chat about with his parents. Most men are uncomfortable about being this unguarded with the women in their lives. They also hesitate about talking to their friends because more likely than not, their male friends will turn the subject into a big joke. The average family doctor is also unlikely to encourage such conversations. In short, unless a man consults with a sex therapist, he may well continue to be confused and unsure of how to handle his erection, which he probably thinks of as having a mind of its own.

Guys with PE may spend a fair amount of time thinking about their issues; they have usually heard guys talking about pleasing women and finding ways of lasting longer; and they have read a book or two looking for suggestions. Here are some of the most common ways in which a guy may try to handle his ejaculation concerns.

He may become very proficient at oral sex or other forms of lovemaking in an attempt to satisfy a woman.

When a man has PE, there are always two separate issues: (1) his being able to last longer and (2), the woman's satisfaction. I firmly believe that even with the worst-case PE scenario, there is no reason why a woman can't have a good time and an orgasm in bed. You just need to be creative. If he wants to satisfy you, he may work really hard at learning new and better ways to use his mouth and hands to give you pleasure. I've known guys who have become so accomplished at massage, for example, that they rival any professional. A man like this may try to satisfy you before he ejaculates, all the while making certain that his penis makes absolutely no contact with your body. This doesn't improve the PE situation because all this body contact usually will make him even more excited so that he will ejaculate within seconds of penetration. Some men will take the opposite approach. Once they have ejaculated, they then concentrate on giving their partners pleasure.

He may secretly masturbate one or more times before he has sex.

Although masturbation may slow down his arousal, and he should indeed be able to maintain his erection for a longer period of time, this is not something I recommend. The woman he is with, for example, may have a sense that his passion or desire for sex is always a little on the diluted side. This method is one that young men with short refractory periods typically tell each other about. Masturbating before sex also isn't going to work for men who have a difficult time getting a second erection within a twenty-four-hour time frame. A more important issue is that masturbating before sex can work against the man's long-term goals. Without realizing it, he is continuing to condition and train himself to ejaculate quickly rather than doing something that will help him learn to last longer. This is also true any time a man masturbates quickly.

He may always plan on having sex more than once.

Some guys automatically assume that in order to satisfy a woman they will need to make love twice in a row. They depend on that second erection to give them more time to satisfy their partners. Again, this works better with younger men who can count on being able to reach a second erection within a short period of time. Men who are able to do this can sometimes be very good lovers. I once had a relationship with a very sexy guy. He regularly lasted not much more than two minutes, but then he would get another erection and be able to have sex for a much longer time. We used to joke about it. He'd say, "Don't worry, this won't take long." I would joke back and say, "That's okay. I have a short attention span." I enjoyed having sex with him because I could tell he liked it. He would use very stimulating positions and get really aroused and make wonderful noises when he ejaculated. In this instance I was okay being with a man who didn't last that long because we both had a good time.

He may try to think about things that will turn him off.

He may try to lessen his arousal by focusing his mind on math problems, money he's earned (or lost), baseball statistics, messy car accidents, his boss, or sex with somebody he finds unattractive.

He may resort to useless products. Does anybody, for example, have any numbing cream?

There are a variety of products sold specifically to reduce sensation in the penis. This is one of the least effective methods of trying to handle PE. One major difficulty is that if any of the cream rubs off on the woman, she will experience the same sensation—or lack thereof. If the man uses a numbing cream, and the woman makes the mistake of attempting oral sex, it goes without saying that it can be a total disaster. A major, although rare, problem is that the lidocaine or prilocaine used in numbing creams can produce dangerous reactions in some people. In a few instances, individuals who used creams with high levels of numbing agents on large areas of their body have actually died. Perhaps the most common drawback to using creams that reduce sensation is that they do just that—reduce sensation. This is simply no fun!

He may visit a doctor who will prescribe one of several selective serotonin reuptake inhibitors (SSRIs). Medications such as Prozac, Paxil, and Zoloft may all help with PE.

These medications are regularly used to treat PE, and yes, they often interfere with ejaculation. Unfortunately, some of these medications also strongly interfere with erections and desire. Effectively using SSRIs to treat PE requires a delicate balancing act. There are men who, working with a doctor, have been able to come up with an appropriate SSRI at the precise dosage needed so that the man is still able to feel desire and maintain an erection, but it's a tricky process. Some MDs advise a low dose taken only on those days when one is expecting to have sex.

I personally am very reluctant to suggest that a man use SSRIs as a way of handling PE. I've known men who have decided to take a drug like Prozac, for example, only to discover that they feel much less desire or become unable to ejaculate at all. This unhappy situation also increases anxiety, which in turn has an impact on sexual behavior, so it can become one vicious circle.

He may deny that he has a problem.

When I was a surrogate, I once had a client whose wife convinced him that as far as sex was concerned, he needed some therapy. He didn't think he was too fast. It didn't take me long to figure out that he lasted about two seconds, but he actually thought he had the opposite problem—that he couldn't get aroused fast enough! He said, "Why don't you wear a sexy outfit to our sessions because it would help me get aroused faster." I told him, "If you get aroused any faster, I'm going to have to open a drive-through window."

Too many men with PE pretend that nothing is wrong and that this is the way sex is supposed to be. Each time a guy like this has sex, he simply hopes that the woman doesn't notice. Because he doesn't acknowledge what's going on, his partner may feel even more uncomfortable about discussing the issue or trying to find solutions.

He may find a partner who doesn't complain and resign himself to bad and boring sex.

This is probably one of the most common ways men deal with PE. I can't even begin to count the number of women I've met over the years who have told me that they have also turned off on sex because their partners are so speedy that it's not worth the effort.

He may read about the squeeze technique and decide to try it.

I personally think the squeeze technique is the kind of sex advice that seems designed to torture women. When learning this method, I was taught that it is best done with the man on the bottom, woman on top. When the man feels he is getting close to ejaculating, he either tells his partner or gives her some kind of signal. The woman is then supposed to hop off and squeeze the head of her partner's penis—hard. I think this is almost an impossible maneuver to accomplish—and trust me, I've tried. I think all it teaches men is the difference between not being aroused and being "too late." Usually by the time the typical guy signals his partner, it's already a lost cause, and the woman ends up feeling as though she is putting her thumb over a garden hose.

He may ask his partner to tug at his testicles.

This is a Masters and Johnson technique. Research showed them that male testicles scrunch up right before ejaculation. So they figured that if you can keep the testicles from doing that scrunch, you can prevent ejaculation. For a woman to tug at a man's testicles, she needs to position herself facing him side by side or under him, and then reach down behind her back and grab his testicles. This works best if you have really long arms or are a trained gymnast. It can be done, but it can also be an uncomfortable turn-off and it doesn't give women much leeway in how they position their bodies for maximum enjoyment. Many men enjoy having their testicles tugged, but it rarely prevents ejaculation. In fact, in my experience it may speed up the process.

He may learn about the stop/start technique and decide this is worth a try.

Once again, the woman is on top. When the man feels he is getting close, he signals his partner and she stops moving. When his arousal level goes down, he signals her that it's okay to start moving again. As far as I'm concerned, this is more on track as a method, and it could help PE since it is at least teaching a man how to gauge his arousal levels. This technique will not work with men with extreme cases of PE because they ejaculate too quickly.

CAN PE BE "CURED"?

The typical guy with PE issues desperately wants to figure out a way to solve his difficulties. I always remember one of the first clients I treated—he ejaculated if you touched his penis. Needless to say, this was very frustrating. Because I was young and inexperienced, I tried to refer him to a more experienced person. But he wanted to remain with me. I gave him a series of exercises and started working with him, but it was apparent that he wasn't doing his homework. He quit therapy. Two years later he came back, and he was worse off than before. This time he was genuinely motivated and he was cured. This was over twenty years ago. Now he's fine and can last as long as he wants. I still talk to him and he confided in me that when he returned to me as a client, he had been so depressed by his ejaculation issues that he felt close to suicidal.

PE can really play havoc with a man's sense of self-esteem. I always remember a client who introduced himself saying, "My name's Ivan, like 'Ivan the Terrible.'"

"Don't worry," I told him. "You've come to the right place. We're going to turn you into 'Peter the Great.'" And we did!

With PE, the guy's attitude is everything.

My friend Kim once went to bed with a guy with PE who blamed her for all his sexual shortcomings. When she tried to talk to him about his feelings, he became defensive and angry, telling her that he had satisfied dozens of women and that if she had problems with how long he lasted (about thirty seconds) maybe it was because he found her so unattractive that he wanted to get it all over with. He was completely shut down and refused to deal with his sexuality honestly and openly. He also had very little interest in learning how to satisfy a woman. Every woman needs to know that some men with PE will resent any woman who tries to help them with their sexual issues. In these instances, the guy has bigger problems than PE and women need to be forewarned.

PE AND THE FEMININE RESPONSE

In the lovemaking department, there is something to be said for a lover who is so excited that he can't wait. In fact, the guy with PE can be a real turn-on because of the intensity and enthusiasm of his response. If you want to continue in a sexual relationship with one of these men, you need to remember some things.

You want to be very up front about your sexual needs without pressuring him to do things he can't do just yet. That means it's up to you to be specific about ways that he can bring you to orgasm without intercourse. You want him to relax and get the message that you are excited by him and you want the sexual connection. Whenever you get the chance, tell him how much you are excited by him as a lover.

You want to encourage him to have as much intercourse as possible. Remember, the more time he spends in your vagina, the more confident and relaxed he will become about lovemaking.

You want to be aware that his tendency to ejaculate rapidly can sometimes put you at risk for pregnancy or an STD. I've known women, for example, who have unintentionally gotten pregnant by men with PE. In all these instances, from the woman's point of view, the man was so eager to thrust his erection into her that she didn't even have time to say, "Stop, put on a condom." While I personally don't accept all those stories about the woman who got pregnant because she went swimming in a heated pool into which some guy ejaculated, I do know how easy it is for some women to become pregnant. In short, whenever a woman is about to have sex with a new partner, she needs to consider the possibility that he may ejaculate so rapidly that the situation is out of control almost before it begins.

HELPING A MAN LAST LONGER

PE is my specialty. I have worked with hundreds of men with this issue. In order for a man to get true and lifelong control of the time he lasts before ejaculating, four things have to happen:

1. He has to learn some relaxation techniques. PE is almost always connected to overall body tension. I always, for example, start out by teaching men about breathing and muscle relaxation.
2. He has to locate and exercise his PC muscle in order to learn to relax it. (See page 221 for this exercise.)
3. He has to learn to experience what he's feeling instead of trying to ignore it or push it away.
4. His body has to become more accustomed to a woman's sensual touch, and his penis has to become more accustomed to the sensation of being inside his partner's vagina.

When men came to me as clients, it was relatively easy for me to teach them to last longer because I had their full attention and cooperation. I would give my typical client a homework assignment that included the exercises found on pages 221–222. If you have the guy's cooperation and agreement, this is the way to go.

But what if you have to be more subtle and find ways to make him last longer without his knowing that you are doing it? This is a bit trickier. Instead of coming right out and saying, "I'm unhappy with our sex life and we have to do something about it," it's probably wisest to use the foot-in-the-door approach by making a series of small requests that build on each other. You can say, "There are some things I enjoy and I want to try them with you. These things will help *me* enjoy sex more."

Start your lovemaking by doing some breathing and relaxation exercises together.

Remember that you want him to relax and slow down. Tell him you're into meditation, yoga, or Zen. This isn't so far-fetched because a lot of people are. Before you have sex, lie on your backs together and practice deep breathing and full body relaxation. Relaxation will slow him down and help put him in touch with what he is feeling. This has an extra bonus of helping you relax, which will also heighten your sexual response.

Three special massages

1. Tell him that you are really into massage or that you have a fantasy about working in a massage parlor (even better if you really have these fantasies). Offer to give him a massage. Start on his back before massaging the front of him. Tell him this is all for him! Tell him if he feels a need to ejaculate, he shouldn't hold back. Pay attention to how his body is responding. This is your chance to learn more about his arousal pattern—how quickly he gets erect and with what type of stimulation. Store this information in your brain for future reference. Stimulate him to ejaculation after all these exercises. The ejaculation is his reward for being able to experience stimulation. This is a major point: Many men with PE don't enjoy their ejaculation. In fact, it has become aversive to them. We have to make it rewarding again.

2. If he enjoyed the first massage (and who wouldn't?), one of

the next times you have sex, do another massage, the same as you did before. This time, however, when you are using your hands on the front of his body, start teasing his penis. In other words, massage very slowly and gently near his penis, using a lot of lubrication. Back off whenever he appears to become too aroused. Your goal here is to prolong the process by increasing the length of time he's receiving stimulation to his penis and prolong the time he's erect without ejaculating. When it becomes apparent that he really needs to ejaculate, be enthusiastic about his orgasm. If it is possible, wait an hour or so and tell him you would like to continue his massage. Do the same thing as before. This time, he should be able to stay erect for a longer period of time.

3. When he has started to show some progress in terms of being able to stay erect without ejaculating, offer him a different kind of massage. Start massaging him as you did in the last exercise. This time, however, when it comes to his penis, switch to oral instead of manual stimulation. Remember that men with PE either dread their ejaculation or try to ignore it. With that in mind, encourage him to make a lot of noise when he ejaculates. You have to convey to him that *you* enjoy it when he ejaculates. It's important for him to feel it is acceptable for him to ejaculate; you like it, and in fact you welcome it.

After you've practiced the massage technique, try some reverse psychology: Tell him, "Wow, you get aroused really easily. That's such a turn-on for me because I love that you're excited by me. I'm so turned on, now we can do something for me." Then show him how to do oral sex just the way you like it.

OTHER SUGGESTIONS FOR BRINGING MORE PLEASURE INTO YOUR SEX LIFE

1. Each time you have sex with him, if he's ejaculated quickly, clean up and put him back inside you in a side-to-side position, even if he's flaccid. It's important for him to spend as much time as he can inside your vagina just so he can enjoy and adjust to the sensations. Use plenty of lubrication for this exercise. Here's a good phrase to use: "I feel so close to you when you're inside me that I want that feeling to last as long as possible."

2. Tell him you want to spend an entire day with him, having sex as many times as you can (or an entire weekend if you both have the time to do this). During a session such as this, don't work or allow other distractions. Each successive time you have sex, he will almost inevitably last longer. I've seen this technique work really well because behaviorally it's very reinforcing for him to last longer and longer each time.

3. To make certain that you have sexual enjoyment, you may have to change the typical sexual script, which goes something like this: The guy goes down on the woman first to show her he's a good guy. Then she returns the favor. That means that when they start to have intercourse, her arousal level is at about a level 2 on a 1 to 10 scale, and he's ready to ejaculate. Instead, ask him to go down on you first and then start intercourse when you are already aroused (or have even had one or more orgasms). That way, it won't bother you if he comes quickly. Save oral sex for him for after he's already ejaculated and actually needs some stimulation to get started again.

4. Encourage him to slow down in general. Without nagging, see if you can encourage him to eat and walk at a more leisurely

pace. Many guys with PE do everything in a rush. Model an attitude where you take your time and savor the moment. Lose the
clocks and watches when you're having sex, and make sure you set
aside plenty of time so there is no rush.

5. Have intercourse with no pressure on him. Convey to him
that you literally don't care how fast he comes, as long as he prom-
ises to enjoy his ejaculation as much as he can.

SOME ADVANCED EXERCISES

Once your guy is more relaxed about sex and appears open to some
new techniques, you may want to encourage him to try the following exercises. You can tell him that you read that these exercises will
help him last longer. Don't forget to tell him that the reason you
want him to do this is because of how much you love having him
inside you, which I'm sure is true or you wouldn't be willing to put
this much energy into his sexuality.

1. *Repetitive Penetration*: Use the butterfly position. (See page
229 for this position.) Ask him to put lots of lubrication on his
penis, and on your vagina if you need it, and kneel in front of you.
Have him put the head of his penis in your vagina and then pull it
back out. Just let the head stay there without moving. Repeat this.
Each time he inserts his penis, let him practice staying there longer. Don't forget to make sure he eventually ejaculates as positive
reinforcement for his staying in for longer and longer periods of
time.

2. *Stop/Start Technique*: Don't try this until he has some de-
gree of control when you are using manual or oral stimulation.
The stop/start technique works best in the butterfly position.
Once he inserts his penis inside you and begins moving, have him

stop as often as he needs to. The trick is for him to stop well before the point of no return. You can also do this exercise when you are on top; he can tell you when to stop and when to start again.

3. *Music, Music, Music:* Find a piece of instrumental music with a slow beat—something like Ravel's *Boléro*, or even a requiem. Try to match your thrusts to the music.

MANY GREAT LOVERS STARTED OUT WITH PE

It might seem like a lot of work and effort to try to be in a sexual relationship with a man who is too quick, but in my experience, it's been well worth it. Some of the best lovers I know have been men with a history of ejaculating very quickly. A fair number of the men I've treated for PE have gone on to become multi-orgasmic. In fact, the men who were the quickest to learn multiple orgasm techniques were the ones who initially ejaculated very rapidly. In my experience, a guy with PE starts off with a definite advantage because he is usually enthusiastic about sex. His eagerness earns him high marks in the lovemaking department. Most of the guys I've known with PE had high energy and lots of passion, which to me are the most important ingredients for good sex.

3

The Guy with Erection Issues

Many sexually active women will be able to relate to the following scenario:

You are in bed with a guy, let's call him Joe. You are both naked, lying on your sides facing each other. Joe's hands and mouth are all over you, and from his breathing, he seems very excited. He reaches down to touch your genitals, and you do the same with his. That's when you notice it: Not only is Joe not erect, he's limper than a silk scarf on a steamy summer day. You are at a loss about what to do next. From the noises he is making, you would have been willing to bet that he was rock hard. You wonder if maybe he hasn't noticed that he's not erect. Is that even possible? Should you tell him? You consider performing oral sex on him, but then you rethink that impulse. Suppose you go down on him, and he still doesn't get erect? How embarrassing! What would you do next? He saves you having to make a decision because he rolls over on top of you and begins to try to stuff his non-erect penis into your vagina. You don't think this is going to work, but you don't want to discourage him. Once again, you consider saying something, but what? Nothing seems appropriate. You wish there were an etiquette book of advice for just such circumstances. You had been very aroused when you took off your clothes, but that feeling has pretty much disappeared and been replaced by anxiety. What is going on, anyway? You wonder if it is something about you that is turning him off. Maybe it's all the garlic in the shrimp scampi you had for dinner; maybe he's noticed the cellulite on your thighs; maybe your breasts are a little less firm than they should be. Could it be any of those things? You wonder how long he will keep trying. You feel as though you are both pretending that everything is all right, when you both know that it isn't. You wish he would say something; you're still afraid to utter a word because he might take it the wrong way. This is no fun!

What do you do when the man in your bed is having problems getting an erection? What can you say? What should you think? What are the reasons? The scenarios in which a man's erection falters are many and far-reaching. Here is some of what you need to know.

When a guy is unable to get an erection, it is formally referred to as erectile dysfunction, or ED, and it is broken down into two main categories: lifelong (or primary) and acquired (or secondary).

Lifelong or primary erectile dysfunction, which is quite rare, means that the man has never, ever, been able to have an erection, under any circumstances whatsoever. In almost all instances of lifelong ED, there is an underlying organic cause, although, for the purposes of treatment, secondary psychological factors may need to be taken into account. If you should become romantically involved with a man who has lifelong ED, he needs sophisticated medical treatment. However, from my experience, I feel comfortable in saying that even the most sexually active woman will rarely, if ever, meet a man who has never had an erection. I know I haven't. However, I personally have known men who were able to have erections when they masturbated or when they were alone, but who were never able to have an erection with a woman or through intercourse. The treatment for these men tends to include psychological as well as medical support.

Acquired or secondary erectile dysfunction, on the other hand, is fairly common; it describes a situation in which a man begins his life as a sexually active male with no erection issues. Then, something—physical, psychological, behavioral, or a combination of all three—happens to change this and the guy starts having either occasional or chronic difficulties. I think it's safe to say that a sexually active woman will almost certainly meet a man who falls into this category. I have seen reports that as many as twenty to thirty million men in the United States have some level of erectile difficulties. Incidents of ED increase as a man ages; therefore, if a woman is having sex with more mature men, it is likely that she will find herself in bed with a man who is having difficulty becoming fully erect. In fact, it is estimated that as many as 50 percent of all men between the ages of forty to seventy will experience some level of ED. I have seen information that indicates that 40 percent of all men in their forties and 70 percent of all men in their seventies are challenged by ED. The popularity of erection enhancement drugs such as Viagra, Cialis, and Levitra certainly confirms this.

Just about every woman I know has been with a man with ED, but until recently it was one of those subjects about which people rarely spoke, except in almost derogatory terms, with snide comments along the lines of "the guy couldn't get it up" or a more polite and almost shameful-sounding whisper, "he was impotent with me." Now ED is finally out of the closet, probably thanks in large part to all those ads for erection enhancement drugs.

Let's state *two* simple facts so that readers can see and remember them.

1. Just as not all women are able to have orgasms whenever they want them, not all men are able to have erections on demand.

It doesn't mean that the guy is a bad person or fatally flawed. All it means is that he is human and not a machine.

2. Just because he doesn't have an erection doesn't mean that he doesn't feel desire. Many women assume, incorrectly, that the absence of an erection means that the guy isn't interested in having sex with them. This is usually not the case. Desire, a product of hormones and emotions, by itself doesn't cause an erection.

SO, WHAT DOES CAUSE ED?

When the man in a woman's bed is unable to get an erection, she typically wants to know why. She wonders, "Is it something physical?" or "Is it all in his head?" Most experts now agree that chronic cases of ED tend to have an underlying organic component.

The most common organic reasons associated with ED include:

Cardiovascular conditions such as heart disease and hypertension
Diabetes
Alcohol consumption
Prescription medications, including common medications prescribed for hypertension, depression, anxiety, and even pain (Some experts believe that as many as 25 percent of all cases of ED are connected to the side effects of prescription medication.)
Illegal/recreational drugs
Hormonal abnormalities
Peyronie's disease (This condition makes the penis curve to one side. It is caused by scar tissue, which in turn hinders blood flow.)
Prostate problems (These include benign enlargement and infections, as well as cancer.)

The most common psychological issues associated with ED include:

Depression
High levels of stress
Generalized anxiety (worries about life, work, money, etc.)
Specific anxiety (high levels of performance anxiety)
Guilt about having sex (he thinks it's wrong—and his penis
    agrees)
Social anxiety disorders (shyness)
Fear of intimacy
Relationship problems

From my own personal experience in working with men with ED, I have observed that there are often both physical and psychological components. A man, for example, might have spent weeks trying to get a particularly attractive woman into his bed. On the night when it finally happens, he is so nervous that he drinks a little bit too much. The effects of the alcohol and the nervousness working together may be enough to give him problems with his erection. This is a sensitive guy who remembers this experience as a real "failure." From that day forward, whenever he is about to go to bed with a woman, he remembers what happened and he feels anxious. He knows that his erection could go down because of anxiety, and it sometimes does.

BEHAVIOR ALSO PLAYS A ROLE

Let's not forget that behavior is sometimes the predominant reason for ED. Here are some examples of situations in which behavior is involved.

He thinks his penis should work like a mechanical tool.

A young guy, for example, may start out with a penis that is unstoppable. Everything turns him on; nothing turns him off. That's how he expects his penis to behave. On those days when he doesn't have sex, he masturbates in the morning and sometimes in the evening as well. A sex machine, that's how he sees himself. Then one Friday night, after having worked a fifty-plus-hour week that involved travel as well as a stressful project for his impossible-to-please employer, he leaves work at six, stops at the gym for a quick forty-five minute workout, races home, and changes his clothes. On the way to pick up his date, he returns a call from his mom who tells him that his beloved grandmother was just hospitalized with what they think is a stroke. It's too late for him to be allowed into the hospital to see her, but he tells his mom that he will meet her there in the morning. He and his date have dinner, a few drinks, and shoot a little pool. Along about midnight, they call it a night. When he gets to his date's house, he and his date both expect to have sex. They start to make out, and he discovers something that he finds impossible to believe: He can't get an erection! He is clueless as to what is going wrong! He honestly can't imagine that his penis could react to stress, fatigue, concerns about his grandmother, or anything else. Impossible! Not *his* penis! Not Old Faithful!

Scenarios like this are extraordinarily common. I once spoke to a guy who told me that he hadn't been able to get an erection the previous weekend, and he was very concerned about it. Saturday morning, he had moved the entire contents of his apartment in a U-Haul truck. Saturday afternoon, he played two games of tennis on an outdoor concrete city court while the temperature soared to over one hundred degrees. By the time he got to his girlfriend's apartment, he was so dehydrated that he could barely walk. Yet he fully expected that once he drank a little bit of Gatorade, he and his girlfriend would spend Saturday night as they usually did, having marathon sex. When he discovered that his penis wasn't cooperating, he was both shocked and concerned.

Many men really want to have penises that respond like mechanical tools and are disappointed by anything else. I once asked a client with ED what his goal was for therapy, and he said, "I want to be able to get an erection even if I don't want one." I'm still trying to figure that one out, although I think his attitude is common: If there was a choice between a magic pill that would create an instant erection and training to learn how to enjoy sex more and please a woman, I'm afraid many men would choose the pill.

He is totally stressed and worried by something that happened that day.

We have all heard about the body's fight or flight reaction to extreme stress. What some of us fail to recognize is how stress causes the body to manufacture higher-than-normal amounts of adrenalin and how that can affect all sexual responses, including erections. It's not unusual for a guy to automatically assume sex is going to help him get rid of all the tension in his body. Unfortunately, sometimes he may be so stressed that his body can't readjust itself that quickly.

He is doing something with his body that is getting in his own way.

Some men consciously or unconsciously tense their bodies, specifically their PC muscles. He needs to know that he can't get an erection with a tensed-up PC muscle.

He is completely out of touch with what he is or isn't feeling, including sensations of arousal.

This is another common scenario. When he was sixteen, he was aroused in about thirty seconds. Now that's he's thirty-five, he thinks nothing has changed, and he goes straight for intercourse without allowing enough time for foreplay and his own arousal.

His penis knows him better than he knows himself.

Let's be honest here. Perhaps the reason he can't get an erection is that unconsciously he believes the relationship isn't good for him. Maybe he's just plain angry at his partner and his penis is responding. So why does he continue to try to have sex under these conditions? Maybe he feels he has something to prove; maybe he's just plain stubborn.

He is trying to have sex after a heavy meal.

Many couples have to make the decision about whether it's food first or sex first. Heavy meals put additional stress on the body. In fact, the American Heart Association recommends that heart patients wait one to three hours after eating before having sex.

He's a smoker.

The number one behavioral factor implicated in ED is definitely smoking because it plays havoc with the small blood vessels in the body, including the ones that bring blood into the penis. Experts agree that smoking is a major risk factor in the development of ED.

He rides his bike regularly.

As if the world wasn't difficult enough, there is a fair amount of research that indicates that riding a bicycle, particularly if the guy is using one of those hard narrow seats, can cause injuries, which, in turn can lead to erectile dysfunction.

WOMEN'S REACTIONS TO ED

How a woman responds to being with a man who has erection difficulties depends upon a variety of factors. If you are fifty-something, and the husband with whom you have shared twenty good years of sex starts having problems with his erection, you are obviously going to respond differently than the twenty-two-year-old who is in bed with a man she recently met. I have found women in their thirties and beyond more understanding of ED than women in their twenties. In fact, I did a survey recently in one of my college classes and discovered that the young women who responded had very little tolerance or understanding about male performance anxiety or problematic erections. This surprised me because I thought that women in their twenties today were better informed than women in my generation were and that these young women would say, "Hey, I have plenty of time for this guy to get it together," and that the older woman would say, "I haven't got that much time left. I can't waste it." But obviously it doesn't work that way.

By and large, couples who are in long-term sexually active relationships tend not to get as concerned about erection issues. If the relationship is intimate and good, and the couple retains the ability to work and play together, it's easier to get past erection issues.

Let's look at a few typical relationships in which the woman is concerned about a man's faltering erection.

Barbie and Geoff

Barbie and Geoff are on their sixth date. Geoff has been pushing for sex since the second date, but Barbie held him off, saying she wanted to get to know him better. They are now on the same page and Barbie is as eager as he is. When they start kissing and taking off each other's clothing, Geoff seems excited and Barbie can feel his erection pressing against her, but almost as soon as he lies down next to her, it disappears. Barbie starts to perform oral sex on him, but even that doesn't seem to coax an erection out of his shrinking penis. Geoff kisses Barbie on the head and says, "Let's give it a rest and try later. It's not you. Sometimes this happens when I'm nervous." What should Barbie think?

Barbie should accept Geoff's explanation. It's very common for a man to have difficulties the first few times he is with a new woman. It usually doesn't mean anything more complicated. In some ways Barbie should be flattered. Geoff is a little nervous because he likes her and he cares about what happens between them in bed. It's also good that Geoff acknowledges and is aware of his pattern. He knows that he needs to relax and stop pressuring himself to perform. I've known many men who have difficulties the first few times with any new woman. Usually, once they get over the hurdle, they are fine from that point forward.

Maggie and Keith

When Maggie met Keith, they were both in their early forties and the sex was terrific and stayed that way until they got married two years later. About a year after the wedding, however, Keith began to have problems with his erection. At first he blamed it on fatigue, so instead of having sex spontaneously at night whenever they were in the mood, they began to schedule appointments to have sex on weekends when they were both less tired. That worked for a while, but now Keith is having difficulty with his erections even when he is rested. Keith continues to want to try to have sex, but Maggie is beginning to worry. Maybe marriage and sex don't mix, at least not for her and Keith. Maybe Keith isn't attracted to her anymore. What does Maggie need to know?

Maggie needs to know that now that Keith is in his midforties, he may well be one of the millions of men whose erections are no longer reliable. The first thing to suggest is that he visit his doctor and possibly a urologist to see if they can find an underlying medical reason for what is happening. The fact that Keith continues to want to try to have sex indicates that he still feels desire even if his erection isn't immediately responding. Once Keith receives a clean bill of health, this is an instance when a medication such as Viagra might make all the difference. Maggie should also relax and put less emphasis on Keith's erection.

Madeleine and Greg

Madeleine is falling in love with Greg, whom she thinks is one of the nicest men she has ever met. One of the things she likes most about him is that he is so affectionate; they spend hours touching and making love. One of the things she likes least about him is that they never have actual intercourse. Greg informed her on their third date that he was "impotent," as he put it. He said that after his ex-wife left him for another man, he became clinically depressed and could no longer get an erection. When he visited a psychiatrist, he was given Prozac, an SSRI, which can contribute to erectile dysfunction. Now he feels much less depressed, but he still can't get an erection, and he's pretty upset about it. He has changed medication, but he continues to have problems. Greg is able to ejaculate without an erection, but he doesn't even try to penetrate Madeleine's vagina. What is going on?

Greg is caught in a cycle, which, unfortunately, is all too common for men who are trying to find a way to treat depression without jeopardizing their sex lives. Men I've known who have been in this position need to be very clear with their prescribing doctors about what is going on, and they have to be willing to be patient. In Greg's case, he still feels desire and he is able to ejaculate, which is a good thing. Even more important, he hasn't given up and is trying to find a solution. This all bodes well for his situation improving. I've seen many clients like Greg. It's almost as if his body got lazy and stopped getting erections because he can ejaculate without one. Greg sounds like the perfect candidate for sensate focus. (See sensate focus exercise on page 223.)

Karen and Bob

Karen and Bob have been in a relationship for over a year, and since the first time they had sex, Bob has been challenged in the erection department. The primary difficulty is that Bob loses his erection soon after penetration. From Karen's point of view, the problem is that Bob tries to have sex too often and keeps trying even when his erection falters. The problem from Bob's point of view is that he needs to take Viagra. What's going on?

When a man is able to get an erection, but then loses it soon after penetration, the cause could be:

Psychological: He suffers from anxiety or performance pressure.

Behavioral: He is trying to have sex too soon after his last orgasm and isn't allowing for a long enough refractory period.

Physical: He might have a condition known as a *venous leak*, which means the erection cannot be maintained because the valves at the base of the penis are damaged and can no longer prevent blood from leaving. A venous leak can be caused by an injury, but it is more likely associated with the aging process.

If Bob is a younger man, then I would suspect that the reason he loses his erection is due to either performance anxiety or not allowing for a long enough refractory period.

Bob should start out by visiting a urologist to rule out a venous leak. It sounds like he needs a full diagnostic workup. In the meantime, both Bob and Karen need to develop a more relaxed attitude about sex and take the emphasis off his erections.

LET'S GET PRACTICAL

When a woman cares for a man with erection issues, she typically wants to know what, if anything, she can do. Here are some suggestions:

Get a better read on what's going on.

When you are with a man who has erection issues, my first suggestion would be to get a handle on whether the problem is primarily physical (he can't have an erection under any circumstances), primarily psychological, primarily behavioral, or a combination of all three. The easiest way to figure out whether a man can have an erection is to determine whether he has nighttime and/or morning erections. Normal healthy men have partial or full erections at about ninety-minute intervals during their sleep cycles. If a man wakes up at the tail end of a sleep cycle, he will usually have a morning erection. So the first thing a woman wants to know is whether he has nighttime erections (also called NPT—nocturnal penile tumescence) or wakes up with a morning erection. If he does, his body is capable of getting an erection. This is good news! If he can get an erection in his sleep, he should be able to get one at some other time.

Other things you should notice: If he can't get an erection at all, with any kind of sexual activity, then his issues are probably going to be physical. If he is able to get and keep an erection with manual or oral stimulation, but loses it when he attempts penetration, this is most likely to be psychological and performance anxiety.

Have a real conversation with him about his erection.

Choose a time and place when it's least threatening and doesn't appear as though you are demanding sex or a better performance. This can sometimes work best when you are having dinner or a quiet conversation—nowhere near a bedroom. Tell him that you've noticed that he is having some issues and say that you want to make sure that it's not something you are doing or not doing. Tell him that you love having intimate contact with him even when he doesn't have an erection and that you don't want to lose that, but that you have sensed he isn't happy with the quality of his erections. Try not to make demands. Here are some things that you should *not* say: "Why don't you ever get it up?" "If you don't get it up soon, I'm out of here!" In fact, I would suggest that you not make any references to "getting it up."

I met a woman years ago who used to complain to all her friends that her husband wasn't having sex with her. At parties, she would drink too much and follow him around demanding to know whether he was going to "get it up" that evening. She actually said things like "Well, you'd better!" She was quite beautiful, and the details behind her marriage would always surprise people. They weren't surprised, however, when the marriage split up. This woman can serve as a role model of how not to have conversations about sex with a man.

What you want to do is remind your guy how attractive he is and how much you love touching him and being touched by him. Act as though not having perfect erections every time is the most normal thing in the world—because it is. Once you have laid the groundwork for talking about his erections, you can discuss it again in the future. Here are some of the things that should be said in conversations you have with him.

1. The most important thing to talk about is whether he has visited a doctor to make certain that he doesn't have any physical issues. Remember that many men resist seeing a doctor until they are pushed. If he doesn't know it already, remind him that there are medical problems as well as medications that affect erections. The list of medications that affect sexual activity is long and far reaching. One woman recently told me that her sexual partner had more difficulty with erections after taking an NSAID (nonsteroidal anti-inflammatory drug) for a sports injury. I had never heard that before—yet, sure enough, when I searched on the Internet, I found some information indicating that they might be implicated in some cases of ED.

2. If you're going to get the most out of this relationship, you're going to need to know something about his sexual history. The only way to do that is to ask him. You want to know if his sexual behavior has changed in the last few years or even months. Is it any different

with you than it is with anybody else? Does he have fewer issues when he masturbates? You also want more history about how his erections have functioned in past relationships. Past performance is often the best predictor of future performance.

3. Ask him about his masturbation and/or porn habits. If you're sleeping together, this really isn't all that personal. What you are trying to do is identify his strengths, not his weaknesses. If watching a certain kind of porn (nothing too disgusting or kinky) gets him hard, tell him that you are willing to go with it (if, indeed, you are). The idea is to use whatever you can find in his history to help make sex better for both of you. Example: If you discover that he finds it easier to get hard by masturbating, suggest that masturbation become part of your foreplay. He can masturbate before he attempts penetration, or he can keep his hand on his penis while he is in you. This, by the way, works best in the butterfly position. (See butterfly position on page 229 and butterfly variation #2 at the end of this chapter.)

IMPORTANT! Pay careful attention to his attitude toward his erection issues or toward having a conversation about them. Ideally he should react honestly and realistically and have some kind of awareness about what is going on. If he gets angry or seems to have a total lack of awareness, these would be red flags for me about whether or not the two of you could find a way to have a satisfying and intimate relationship.

MEDICATIONS, DEVICES, AND OTHER INTERVENTIONS

If your guy goes to a doctor, he may well return with a prescription for a medication. We've all seen the endless advertisements on TV so we probably already know that the most common oral medications currently used to treat ED are selective enzyme inhibitors such as Viagra, Levitra, and Cialis. These are prescription drugs, which can typically be used up to once a day. They all have a high success rate. A guy taking these medications should discuss them thoroughly with his doctor because there are some existing medical conditions that may preclude their use. An MD will also make sure that the man is not taking certain other medications such as nitrate drugs and alpha blockers. A man's doctor should take a thorough medical history and give him a complete physical before prescribing any of these drugs. This is important! He shouldn't be getting these drugs from any questionable sources without adequate medical advice and supervision.

What we all need to remember about these medications is that they don't work without sexual stimulation and arousal. This is not a situation in which a guy pops a pill and immediately gets an erection. He still needs to feel desire and become aroused. Viagra is usually prescribed to be taken thirty minutes to one hour before a man hopes to have sex. Levitra is taken an hour before. Viagra and Levitra are both usually effective for up to two hours after they are taken. Cialis has a much longer half-life and can work for up to thirty-six hours, which allows for more spontaneity. The most common side effects of these selective enzyme inhibitors include facial reddening, nasal congestion, and indigestion. The first time you have sex with a man who is taking one of these medications, you may be shocked at how flushed he becomes, so don't be alarmed.

Each man should discuss the medication options with his doctor. He may want to get a limited supply of each of these medications and try them one at time to see which works best for him and produces the fewest side effects. Also, while these medications do work much of the time, don't be surprised if they aren't a magic cure-all. You may still want to use some of the positions and techniques I suggest to enhance his erection and your love-making.

There are other options to help improve erections. A man should discuss all of these with his urologist.

Testosterone: Testosterone can help increase desire, if that is the underlying issue, but it's debatable whether it has any real effect on erections.

Injectable Medications: There are self-injectable substances that cause penile arteries to dilate. Most men who use this method say the injections are relatively pain-free and find this a useful treatment, but others are squeamish about this treatment because it requires an injection into the penis itself.

Urethral Suppositories: These are tiny pellets that a man places down his urethra. They contain medication that also dilates the arteries. These work better for some men than others.

Vacuum Erection Device: This is a cylinder into which a man places his penis. When he pumps the air out of the cylinder, it pulls blood into the penis, causing an erection. This device is typically used with a rubber ring that is positioned around the base of the penis. This helps maintain the erection.

Penile Implants: There are now several varieties of penile prostheses. Getting one requires a surgical procedure, but many men say that it is well worth the effort.

SOME SUGGESTIONS FOR WORKING AROUND ED

I don't believe in giving up on the guy with ED. Having said that, I also realize that nothing is going to happen unless he is able to relax about what is or isn't happening with his penis. It's important to convince a man that he can have intercourse even if he doesn't have a full erection (or even an erection at all). I remember telling one of my clients this. He said, "Trying to have sex without an erection is like trying to shoot pool with a rope." It's a funny statement, but it's not true. A guy can still be intimate and connected and feel his partner's vagina even if his penis is not that hard. Here are some suggestions that have worked for me with men of all ages whose erections were challenged.

Develop a more relaxed, easygoing attitude about erections.

Even if performance anxiety is not the cause of ED, it's often part of the total picture of what's going on. Performance anxiety is most likely to occur when a guy is with a new woman and doesn't feel totally comfortable or at ease, but it can happen whenever a man feels that he is being watched, judged, or pressured to perform. If you are in bed with a guy, we have to assume that it's because you like him for reasons other than the firmness of his penis. Keep that in mind and try to be accepting of the whole person. The best attitude for you: If he has an erection, great. If he doesn't, we can still have fun in bed.

Don't assume responsibility for his erections.

A woman can easily become tense and anxious herself when she is with a man who is having erection issues. Frequently, she immediately assumes that she is somehow at fault in the situation—"He's not having an erection because he doesn't find me desirable." "He's not having an erection because I hate oral sex." "He's not having an erection because I asked him to go to the store last week and now he thinks I'm too demanding." This kind of thinking is ridiculous and doesn't mesh with what we know about the male sexual response.

Have sex when you are both rested.

Sex is a great way to say "good morning"! I've known so many men whose erections are better when they first wake up. Even if morning sex isn't your thing, do it a few times just to see if his erections are firmer at that time. If they are, but you really can't get into morning sex, start having sex later in the day, but suggest that you both nap together first to see if his erections improve when he is more rested. Typically, men with ED have the most difficulty when they are tired.

Get comfortable about touching and caressing his penis when it is soft.

Men are often uncomfortable about having a woman touch their penis except when it is hard, and many women have very little experience in touching or performing oral sex on a penis that is soft. Try to get over this. Remember that his penis can experience pleasure whether it is hard or soft. Some men simply require more stimulation, so don't become nervous or anxious if he doesn't become hard within seconds of your starting oral sex, for example.

Don't be afraid to incorporate masturbation into your foreplay.

If masturbation works to give him a better erection, don't be shy about sharing masturbation with each other. It can become even sexier and more intimate if you kiss and make lots of eye contact.

Become more familiar with different levels of erections.

Think of erections on a 1–10 scale with 1 representing no erection and 10 being diamond-cutter hard. As blood flows into a penis, it gets warmer and harder. Levels 2, 3, and 4 represent a penis in which this is happening; it is filling with blood and getting harder and harder. Levels 5–10 represent different degrees of rigidity. At a 10, a penis gets that spring-back quality. You can have sex with him when his penis is only beginning to fill, but you should use the side to side position. For levels 5, 6, 7, the butterfly position works best. For levels 8–10, you can pretty much have intercourse in any position the two of you want.

TECHNIQUES THAT I'VE USED

When I was working with clients, there were some techniques that I found made a big difference. Here are some of my suggestions:

Oral sex can work wonders.

Most men appreciate oral sex. In my experience (which, by now, I'm sure you have figured out is substantial), there is no such thing as too much oral sex. It goes without saying, however, that the oral sex you do have with your partner will be most effective, in terms of his erection, if you really enjoy doing it. The more you like it and convey that you like it, the more relaxed he'll be. If you don't enjoy oral sex all that much, but are happy to do it because it works to get him erect, then try a combination of oral and manual manipulation. Switch back and forth or use your hand on the shaft of his penis and your mouth on the head.

Here is a good exercise for oral sex: Lie down on your side and have the man kneel next to you. Prop your head up with one hand and lick his penis on the underside so that you are "going up" on him (as opposed to down). Gravity will help him in this situation. If it's comfortable for you, he could also straddle your chest so you can use the same movement.

Check out PC muscle relaxation.

Some men don't get erections because of a very simple reason: The PC muscle is in an almost-constant state of tension. In fact, one of the ways that erection enhancement medications work is to relax the PC muscle. To help him learn how to relax his PC muscle by himself, suggest that he lie on his back. Slowly lick and suck his penis, conveying no sense of psychological pressure or expectation. Cup your hand under his balls. Every time his PC muscle tightens up (indicated by his testicles twitching), stop the stimulation until he relaxes it.

POSITIONS TO USE / POSITIONS TO AVOID

If a man has erection difficulties, there are two positions that I wouldn't advise using. One is the straight missionary position. It's too stressful for a guy to try to support his body weight with one arm while he attempts to insert a less-than-firm penis with his other hand. The second position to avoid is the female superior position. Psychologically, this can make the guy feel overwhelmed and exacerbate the problem. Physically, even if he is able to insert his penis, because of gravity, it's likely to fall out. (We don't want to experience any more fallout than necessary.)

Here are some positions that work even when the penis is mostly flaccid:

Side by Side Scissors Position

Use lots of lubrication on both his penis and your vagina. Your man lies on his right side. You lie on your back perpendicular to him. Scoot together so that your genitals are touching. Put your right leg between his legs and your left leg on top of his left leg.

Encircle the base of his penis with your index finger and thumb. Line up his penis along the opening of your vagina. Use your other hand to push the shaft of his penis into your vagina. The head will follow.

Press your pelvises together. Close your eyes and focus on the sensations of warmth and moisture. To move, grind your pelvises together so that his penis stays inside.

Talk to each other, caress each other, and look into each other's eyes. Avoid coughing or laughing because the movement will cause your PC muscle to push his penis out of your vagina. Continue this for as long as you want. Who knows, maybe when his penis gets in there, it will harden enough for him to begin thrusting.

Butterfly Position Variation #1

(The butterfly position is my favorite under just about all circumstances. See page 229 for the basic butterfly position.)

Start out by putting lots of lubrication on both his penis and your vagina. Lie on your back and tilt your pelvis so your legs are spread up in the air. Your guy should kneel in front of you. Make sure that you have used plenty of lubrication. When you are trying to insert a semi-erect penis in the butterfly position, here's what to do: Line the penis up with your vaginal opening so the head of the penis is against your clitoris. Put your finger and thumb around the base of his penis and gently squeeze as though your fingers are forming a cock ring. Then push the shaft into your vagina with your thumb. The head will follow. (Yes, you are reading that correctly—the shaft goes in before the head.) If the penis is very large, this may not work. In that case, you need to put the head in first and then use a combination of sucking it in with your PC muscle and grabbing the base like a cock ring and pushing.

Now the man thrusts slowly, making sure that his penis doesn't come completely out of the vagina.

Some of the side benefits of this position: The guy gets a good view of his penis going in and out, and from this angle when he looks down, he appears hard. Psychologically, this, combined with the male superior position, can help enhance his sense of control. This is also a good position for you to stimulate your clitoris in order to increase your own arousal. Also, he can periodically remove his penis and add more lubrication and run it up and down your vaginal lips and over your clitoris.

Butterfly Position Variation #2

Once again, get into the butterfly position. If he gets a stronger erection with masturbation, have him stimulate himself while you do the same for yourself.

Lie on your back and put your legs up. Have him kneel between your legs and put lots of lubrication on both of you. He can continue to masturbate while he rubs his penis on your vagina. The difference between this and the last exercise is that he keeps his hand on his penis and continues to push it in and out of your vagina. For him, it's like masturbating and having intercourse at the same time. Wow! That's a turn-on!

Bottom Line: Just because a guy isn't fully erect doesn't mean he can't be a terrific lover. Honest!

4

He Never Seems to Ejaculate!

Brenda is having sex with Eric, and it's turning into a very emotional experience. Unfortunately, the emotion Brenda is experiencing is closer to anger than it is to passion. Here's why: Brenda and Eric have been having sex for almost two hours. They have done it standing up and sitting down. She has been on top of him, and she has been underneath him. Her legs have been over his shoulders, and they have been wrapped around his back. Brenda performed oral sex on Eric for so long that she wonders if her neck will ever recover, not to mention her jaw. They even spent a long twenty minutes on the couch so that Eric could watch a porn video on the living room television while Brenda knelt in front of him, her tired jaw bobbing up and down. Eric has now been on top of her for a full thirty-five minutes. He is very vigorous, and with every thrust, her head makes contact with the headboard and the "swoosh-whack" sound is driving her nuts.

Brenda wants to be a good sport about what's going on, but she is tired and dry and she has cramps in her legs. She wouldn't mind so much, but she has had sex with Eric enough times to have figured out that no matter what Eric does, he will not have an orgasm, and he will not ejaculate. What's going on here? Brenda has been going out with Eric for five months; she likes him and wants to continue the relationship. She likes talking to him and listening to music with him; she likes going to the movies with him and hanging out in his kitchen, watching him cook. Eric is a terrific cook, and when she watches him make pizza from scratch, she feels as though this is somebody she wants to know for the rest of her life. What she doesn't like is having sex for so long that it becomes painful. There are two reasons why Brenda hasn't complained to Eric: She doesn't want to hurt his feelings and she doesn't want to hurt the relationship. Nonetheless, she's beginning to get angry at Eric for being insensitive to how uncomfortable it sometimes is to have sex with him. She wonders why she should have to tell him. Why hasn't he figured it out for himself? And why doesn't he do something about it?

WHAT IS DELAYED EJACULATION?

Delayed ejaculation (or DE) is exactly what it sounds like. It describes a situation in which a man, who is aroused and having penile stimulation, is unable to ejaculate. Men who experience delayed ejaculation are not nearly as common as men who have erection problems or who ejaculate quickly, but if you invite enough men into your bed, I can guarantee that you are going to meet at least one.

Since the guy who has difficulty ejaculating is frequently someone who has no difficulty with erections, he may initially appear to be a super-stud. Therefore, his sexual issues are sometimes overlooked or downplayed. Nonetheless, guys who don't ejaculate are generally very unhappy about their difficulties, even though they may act as though nothing unusual is taking place. I've actually known men who were so embarrassed by their inability to achieve orgasm that they became quite adept at "faking it." More than one woman has told me of having sex with a man as many as five or six times before realizing what wasn't happening.

Over the years, the inability to ejaculate has been given many different names. It's been called male frigidity, retarded ejaculation, ejaculatory incompetence, and inhibited ejaculation. The current name that is frequently used is male orgasm disorder. This name creates a certain amount of theoretical confusion because orgasm and ejaculation are not exactly the same. Orgasm is the full body release that includes rapid heart rate along with a mental and emotional sense of release or pleasure. Ejaculation is the part of orgasm that happens when the PC muscle spasms and semen is released from the penis.

I always like to remind women that it is possible for a man to have the feelings of an orgasm without ejaculating; in other words a man could be having an orgasm even though no semen comes out. In fact, there are men who voluntarily choose not to ejaculate. They may do this for religious or cultural reasons. In some Asian cultures, it's considered preferable if a man doesn't ejaculate very often. They believe that men should have nonejaculatory orgasms because ejaculating depletes your "chi," or vital energy or essence. They believe that a man is more powerful if he doesn't ejaculate. In these cultures, many men make a conscious choice to hold back even though they are fully able to ejaculate. This is a learned skill, and I have done a good deal of work in this country teaching men exercises that will make it possible for them to experience orgasms without ejaculating until they choose to do so.

For the purposes of this chapter, however, we are specifically referring to men who are unable either to ejaculate or to experience the full body release known as orgasm, and I am using the terms interchangeably. There are obviously varying degrees of

DE. The mildest and least disruptive example of DE is the guy who is occasionally unable to have an orgasm when having sex. An extreme example of DE is the man whose only experience of ejaculation is during wet dreams. When most experts talk about DE, they are referring to the man who is unable to ejaculate with a woman during intercourse or oral sex, even though he is able to do so while masturbating, which is the most common DE pattern.

Here are examples of four men who have difficulty ejaculating under different conditions:

Frank's pattern

Frank had an orgasm from intercourse with a woman named Diane on Monday night. He and Diane had sex again on Tuesday and Wednesday, but he was not able to ejaculate. However, early Thursday morning, before leaving for work, he and Diane had sex again; this time he had an orgasm and ejaculated. On Thursday night, Frank had a date with Melanie. He was tired, but not so tired that he didn't want to have sex. Once again, however, he was unable to ejaculate. He didn't do so until Friday evening when he masturbated alone before going to bed. He spent Saturday night with Melanie and they had sex; but once again he wasn't able to have an orgasm or ejaculate. It doesn't take a Ph.D. in sex to realize that Frank doesn't have a serious issue with DE. He is able to have orgasms and ejaculate with a woman; he just can't do it as often as he might like. If Frank wants to ejaculate every time he has sex, he needs to pay more attention to his refractory period. (P.S. If you are sleeping with someone like Frank, and if he is also sleeping with other women, you are going to be totally confused by what is happening in bed.)

Tom's pattern

Tom is a completely different story from Frank. Although he has dated an impressive number of women and is always interested in having sex, he has never ejaculated inside a woman. On two separate, and notable, occasions more than ten years ago, he was able to ejaculate when a woman performed oral sex. Tom, however, is able to achieve orgasms and ejaculation from masturbation, which he does regularly when he is alone. Tom's relationships tend to remain casual; he doesn't talk to any of his dates about his issues with delayed ejaculation and doesn't feel that any of his relationships have been serious enough to warrant a real conversation. And, yes, when Tom has sex with a woman more than a few times, he sort of fakes it so that no questions will be asked. Tom believes that when he is in a committed love relationship with the right woman, they will be able to work things out and he has hopes that his issue will magically disappear.

Jim's pattern

Jim's ejaculatory history is slightly different from both Tom's and Frank's. Jim has had several long-term girlfriends with whom he had enjoyed a great deal of sex without ejaculation or orgasm. Jim, however, has difficulty ejaculating even while masturbating. He says that if he is lucky, he has an orgasm every month or two with masturbation. When Jim is in bed with a woman for the first time, before they have sex, but after she has taken her clothes off, he usually tries to say something that will prepare her for his pattern. He says something along the lines of, "Sometimes I have difficulty having orgasms, so don't be surprised." He doesn't want a woman to reject him because of his ejaculatory issues. He feels there will be less likelihood of this happening if the relationship is more established before he discloses too much. In short, he wants the women he dates to know him and like him before they get the full picture about his difficulties with ejaculation.

Burt's pattern

Burt has still a different issue. He never had any problems with ejaculation until he started taking medication for depression and OCD (obsessive-compulsive disorder). Now, although he still ejaculates, it feels as though it takes an eternity to get there. He is married, and his wife is quite unhappy by how long it is taking him to have an orgasm, but they both recognize the trade-off they are making in terms of his mental health, and for the moment, this is what they both want to do.

WHAT ARE THE REASONS FOR DE?

Although delayed ejaculation usually has its roots in behavioral conditioning or psychological issues, there are also physical problems that will contribute to the pattern.

Possible medical issues that might be implicated in DE

Any man who is experiencing DE should always visit a competent doctor to rule out medical reasons first. Here are some of the medical issues that contribute to DE.

Neurological problems: Diseases such as multiple sclerosis, diabetes, nerve damage, or stroke can affect a man's ability to ejaculate.

Prostate problems: Men who experience delayed ejaculation should be checked by a doctor who can determine whether or not the prostate is involved and prescribe appropriate treatment.

Medications: SSRIs such as Prozac, Paxil, and Zoloft are notorious for causing problems with ejaculation and orgasm. MAO inhibitors also prescribed for depression can have the same effect.

Possible psychological causes of DE

When there are psychological reasons connected to a guy's DE, within the relationship these issues will tend to show up in nonsexual as well as sexual ways. Some experts believe that when a man has DE, there is almost always a psychological component or reason. Here are some of them.

Identifiable trauma: Men who have identifiable traumas will typically have vivid memories of the event. For example, years ago, I had a relationship with a man named Kenneth. He was a good lover and I enjoyed having sex with him, but he never ejaculated. He told me, however, that he had orgasms. It didn't seem to me that he did, but this was before I went to work in a sex clinic, and I wasn't about to argue with him. He gave me a story that I couldn't quite believe, but it was interesting nonetheless: He said that when he was in the army, he had been taken as a POW and that his captors tortured him by showing him pictures that would cause him to get erections. If he did, they would cut him on his penis. This story seemed way over-the-top to me, but if it was true I could certainly understand why something like this would cause a man to tense up during sex and not ejaculate.

Men who are able to connect their issues with ejaculation to a traumatic event often do well with counseling or therapy. I know of one case of a young man who was having sex with his girlfriend in her parents' home when the parents walked in unexpectedly.

He jumped up and ejaculated right in front of them. From that day forward, he had a difficult time ejaculating until he saw a sex therapist and spent some time working through his issues.

Fear of intimacy: Consciously or unconsciously, some men have a deeply held belief that ejaculating inside a woman's vagina signifies making a commitment. These men are simply afraid of too much emotional intimacy with a woman. They can manage the act of intercourse, but when it comes to ejaculation or orgasm, they don't expect anything to happen. A guy like this has issues with trust as well as love and intimacy and if he is going to overcome his difficulties, he will probably need a great deal of psychological support.

Fear of getting a woman pregnant: Dennis, who had a very unhappy childhood, is terrified by the prospect of ever becoming a father himself. He believes that his problems with ejaculation are directly connected to these feelings. Like Dennis, some men are completely aware of this fear; with others, it is so deeply unconscious that it requires some kind of therapy or counseling to uncover.

An underlying or unconscious belief that sex is dirty: If you think sex is dirty, it follows that you are going to believe that if you derive pleasure or satisfaction from it, then you are dirty also. Whether they got this belief from their religious beliefs or from their parents, some men have been deeply indoctrinated with feelings such as these; they can't bring themselves to have so much pleasure from sex that they have orgasms.

Anger: Women who share their beds with men who can't ejaculate often wonder whether anger is an underlying issue. "Does he hate all women, or is it just me?" is the kind of question that is sometimes asked. These women are not alone: Freudian psychoanalysts typically believed that the inability to ejaculate, particularly with intercourse, was caused by repressed anger at women. While I don't agree with this kind of blanket approach, it does seem that at least some men have ejaculatory issues that are connected to a negative view of women.

Obsessive compulsive disorder (OCD): A guy who is obsessive about cleanliness, for example, might have issues with ejaculating in a woman's vagina, or he might have a ritualized sexual pattern that doesn't allow for ejaculation, or he may want to control everything to such a degree that he can't allow himself to ejaculate. Sometimes the man who thinks sex is dirty also has OCD. Unfortunately, some of the medications given for OCD are cited as causing DE, so medical management requires a highly skilled professional.

An unappealing partner: Over a period of years, Jeff grew to actively despise his wife. It reached a point where there was nothing about her that he liked. Nonetheless, Jeff didn't believe in divorce and had very fixed ideas about what a husband should do. Like an automaton, he initiated sex at least once a week. He was able to get an erection because he fantasized about a woman at work. But the fantasy always evaporated too quickly and he couldn't have an orgasm. It's not unusual for a guy to be unable to ejaculate with a specific partner he really doesn't want to be with. The reasons can vary from no longer being attracted to a specific woman to no longer being attracted to any woman. The major issue here, of course, is why a man would cling to a relationship he doesn't really want to have.

Possible behavioral causes of DE

Behavior is frequently a causative factor in DE. Here are some examples:

Practicing a masturbatory style that didn't prepare him for sex with a woman: Does he have a history of masturbating with such a firm, fast, stroke that the vagina cannot duplicate it? This is actually one of the more common reasons why guys have difficulties ejaculating with intercourse. When Doug, for example, started masturbating during puberty, he developed a style that can best be described as beating up his penis. Faster and harder was the only method he knew. Now that he has started having sex with women, however, he has a real issue. He likes having sex, but no way does it give him the stimulation he needs. Doug is one of many, many men for whom this is true, which is one of the reasons why I always recommend that men train themselves to masturbate using a style that more closely resembles vaginal contact. I tell them to start training themselves for slower, more sensual lovemaking by using lubrication and trying to duplicate the way a vagina feels.

Tensing up his PC muscle right before ejaculation: When I was working with a man who wanted to be able to sustain his erection without ejaculation, I would teach him exercises that helped him strengthen his PC muscle so he could put off ejaculation. Guys who don't easily ejaculate have the exact opposite issue from those who ejaculate too quickly. Guys with delayed ejaculation need to learn how to relax the PC muscle so that they will be able to ejaculate. I've known men who used to have premature ejaculations and who were so nervous about the PE returning that they overcompensated by trying to control their ejaculations all the time, and ultimately this backfired (yes, a pun was intended). Many men experience this every now and then when they hold back their ejaculation for such a long period of time that they reach a point where it just isn't going to happen.

Regularly using withdrawal as a form of birth control: Some men have pulled out so many times that they have inadvertently conditioned themselves not to ejaculate. I remember one man I worked with who had been using the withdrawal method for most of his life. He was already in his forties when he came to me because he was unable to ejaculate from intercourse. After several months, he actually got to the point where he could ejaculate within a reasonable time frame of intercourse—fifteen to twenty minutes.

Drinking heavily: It's not unusual for a guy to be unable to ejaculate when he has been drinking too much. What few men realize is that the inability to ejaculate can be a long-term effect of alcohol abuse.

Anticipating his ejaculation well before it is about to happen: Most men start to think about coming when they are around a level 8½ on a 1 to 10 scale. The guy with ejaculation issues may start anticipating it down around level 6. Then he tenses up and starts working at making sure he is going to ejaculate. That puts psychological pressure on him and he tenses up too much, and the more pressured he feels about ejaculating, the more difficult it becomes to do so.

Making the mistake of thinking he is aroused simply because he is erect: A very well-known and experienced sex therapist and researcher named Bernie Apfelbaum used to refer to men with "automatic erections." When he did so he was talking about the kind of guys who seem to be able to get erect from the reverberation of a ceiling fan. The slightest stimulation makes them erect. But despite their erections, these men may not be truly aroused. A guy like this tends to start intercourse with a firm erection, but an arousal level that's only around a 2. They then have the same problem a woman does in trying to catch up.

HOW MEN FEEL ABOUT HAVING DE

Most men are extremely disturbed and upset about having DE, and this feeling goes way beyond the physical frustration of not being able to have orgasms with their partners. Many of them have read the literature on DE. They know, for example, that their masturbatory habits could be implicated as a cause. This information may leave them with feelings of shame or embarrassment, however unwarranted these might be. Sometimes they may have psychological issues, which they realize are connected to the DE. When they meet a new woman, they are frequently embarrassed about her finding out about their issues and they often resist having honest, open conversations.

Typically, the guy with DE wants to know why he is so different from the vast majority of men who, no matter what else is going on, are always able to ejaculate. He wants to know why he was "chosen" for this incredibly difficult sexual pattern. His emotional reaction to DE may cause him to do all kinds of things in bed that work against him.

HOW WOMEN RESPOND

A man who can have sex for hours sounds like every sexy woman's dream, but instead it can sometimes be closer to a nightmare in a category labeled "Be Careful What You Wish For." Delayed ejaculation can be very troubling for a woman for several reasons. Here are some of them:

- On a purely physical level, she may complain, for example, that she doesn't like having sex for hours on end. She often complains that making love becomes a chore instead of a pleasure.
- She may want to get pregnant the old-fashioned way and may not relish the idea of having to consult doctors for advice on how to get sperm from her partner's body into hers.
- It may make her feel insecure, and she may question her

desirability. She may think things like "Maybe he really isn't that into me; maybe he would rather be with somebody else."

- She may view her partner's inability to ejaculate as her own personal failure and think things like "I can't be much of a woman if I can't even bring him to orgasm."
- She may feel frustrated and believe that the sex itself isn't complete without her partner's orgasm.
- She may feel guilty that she is able to have an orgasm and he isn't.
- She may feel that his inability to ejaculate is a barrier to true intimacy. I've heard women say things like "It feels like he doesn't want to be close to me. It feels like he doesn't trust me."
- She may become angry and come to think that her partner is willfully "refusing" to ejaculate or have an orgasm. She may say things like "I swear it feels like he is trying to punish me."
- She may come to view the DE as symptomatic of many other problems within the relationship.

How a woman responds to a man with DE is often very dependent on the nature of the relationship itself. If it's a good relationship, the couple has a better chance of finding ways of resolving their sexual issues. Phoebe, a thirty-eight-year-old woman who is very sexually experienced, told me that DE was a contributing factor in the breakup of her last relationship. She said:

"It wasn't the fact that Stan couldn't have an orgasm that bothered me. What bothered me was that he withheld from me in so many ways. He didn't seem to want to give to me or take care of me. It felt like his inability to ejaculate was one more way for him to show me that he didn't want to be in a relationship with me."

Like Phoebe, some women begin to associate their partners' DE with all the other things that can go wrong in a relationship. Yet there are certainly other women who have been able to build satisfying relationships with men who have DE.

DOES DE EVER GET BETTER?

Sex therapists know that DE is one of the most obstinate male sexual patterns. If there are, for example, deep-seated psychological issues, it's not going to be resolved with a snap of the fingers. However, I also know that tomorrow morning a drug company could announce that a new medication is suddenly available, and DE could become a thing of the past.

In the meantime, if the man in your bed has DE, let's be honest and direct about how likely it is that his difficulties will immediately disappear. If his DE is directly connected to medical conditions or medications, then he needs to first deal with those problems with the support of a medical professional. If his DE seems to be the result of behavior and how he learned to masturbate, then you should be able to use behavioral techniques to change what he is doing. If his DE is directly connected to deeper psychological issues, then in all likelihood, he will need psychological help to overcome his challenges.

With all of this, we need to take other things into account, like his age and his history. For example:

If the man in your bed is still young (in his twenties, thirties, or early forties) and he is able to ejaculate easily with masturbation, the chances are genuinely good that you will both be able to find a creative way to work through his ejaculation issues.

If the man in your bed is relatively young and has ejaculated with intercourse with partners in his past, he will probably be able to do it again with you.

If the man in your bed is in his forties or fifties, has problems achieving an orgasm (even with masturbation), and has never ejaculated with intercourse, the chances that it will spontaneously happen are not good.

If the man in your bed was once able to ejaculate with intercourse, but now he's in his sixties, seventies, or eighties and has severe erection problems combined with ejaculation problems, he will need medical treatment to help deal with his difficulties.

FIXING DE—WHAT NEEDS TO HAPPEN

Make no mistake about it, fixing DE is not a piece of cake—but it can be done. If you care enough about a particular special man to work with him, you need to have a clear sense of what the two of you need to accomplish. For a guy's situation with DE to improve, three things need to happen.

1. He needs to learn to trust his partner at least enough to ejaculate. On some very basic level, if you are without trust, you are never going to be able to have an orgasm with a partner. This is true of both men and women. Men with DE often have trust issues with women in general (and sometimes more so with a specific partner).

2. He needs to get rid of some of his inhibitions and insecurity about sex. Of course, none of us are ever totally without inhibitions or sexual insecurity. But men with DE are often especially inhibited and worried about being judged.

3. He needs to change his masturbatory habits to help his penis become more sensitive to the kind of stimulation that a vagina or a mouth provide. This is one of the most essential elements in changing the pattern of a guy with DE.

THE WOMAN'S ROLE

You probably want to know what you as a woman can do to make it better. How should you think about what you are doing? How should you see your role in the process? Here are some suggestions:

Realize that it's not your problem.

If you are going to have a satisfying relationship with somebody with DE, you have to make sure that you don't let the entire focus of the relationship become whether or not he ejaculates. You can't feel as though you are somehow at fault because he fails to have an orgasm. You can't feel guilty because your vagina doesn't duplicate the stimulation of his hand. We had a saying at the sex clinic where I worked: "People are responsible for their own orgasms. You can't make somebody else have one." Remember that. Also, don't get overly caught up in working on his orgasm. After all, you wouldn't want someone to pressure you to have an orgasm, would you?

Change your script about what it means to have sex.

Most people think sex is over when the man ejaculates. When you're having sex with a guy with DE, that's not how it works. You are either going to have to set clear time limits about how long you can have sex, or decide that sex is over when *you* have had an orgasm. Realize that nothing bad is going to happen to the guy just because he didn't ejaculate. Look at it this way—if he was aroused enough, he would ejaculate and nothing could stop him because it's a reflex. Therefore he's not aroused enough to ejaculate, so he's not aroused enough to have discomfort from the lack of a release.

Find out his sexual history.

If you are in bed with a guy who is experiencing delayed ejaculation, the first thing you want to do is get as much of his sexual history as you can. You want to determine how serious an issue it is, and in order to do that, there are several questions that you need to have answered. Is this something that happens occasionally or is it happening all the time? Has he ever ejaculated in the past, and under what conditions? Has he ever ejaculated while having intercourse with a woman? Is he able to ejaculate from masturbation? Has he ever had wet dreams? The answers to these questions will help you decide whether or not this is a sexual problem you want to tackle.

Get a sense of his attitude.

Strong motivation and a good attitude are essential to a successful outcome. If he seems resigned to his situation or even reluctant to alter the status quo, you are facing an almost insurmountable challenge. But if he is genuinely frustrated by his sexual pattern and really wants to change it, your chances are good that the situation can improve.

MAKE MASTURBATION YOUR FRIEND

Many women are squeamish about male masturbation. They say, "Ycch!" They don't understand its value in working through sexual issues. They say, "Why does he need to play with himself when I'm willing to do it for him?" Women don't like it because it makes them feel as though they are unnecessary. They say, "It's apparent he doesn't need me; he's got himself." If this is your attitude toward masturbation and you truly want to construct a satisfying sexual relationship with a guy who has DE, my best advice is to get over it!

Since many of the behaviors that either created the DE or allowed it to flourish got their start in masturbatory patterns or styles, it stands to reason that we use masturbation to try to shake things up and change things around. The first goal you want to accomplish, for example, is having him masturbate to orgasm while he is with you. Here are some suggestions for doing just that:

Try a simple fix that sometimes works.

Find out how much he masturbates and suggest that he cut way back, particularly on the days before you are supposed to get together. You want him to have a real edge. It sounds unbelievable, but for some men, this in itself is enough to make a real difference.

Masturbate together as part of your lovemaking. (This is an important exercise because it's also a way of increasing his trust, as well as yours.)

Make masturbation a more sensual and intimate experience and include each other in what you are doing. Let him watch you and kiss you and touch you while you masturbate. Do the same for him.

Make love without having intercourse. Lick and kiss his body, for example. Some men enjoy having a vibrator used around or on their penis while they pleasure themselves. Maybe he enjoys having the area around his anus stroked and this will send him over the edge. Or maybe he likes his nipples licked or touched. Sometimes these seemingly small touches can have a big impact, if he can relax enough to allow himself to get to the edge. If you are both masturbating at the same time, make eye contact. Show your support and feelings by kissing, touching, and encouraging each other's pleasure.

When he is masturbating, watch what he is doing and let him watch you.

See if he is doing that hard fast stroke or tensing up his PC muscle. Next time you go down on him, encourage him to change those habits.

Incorporate some sensate focus exercises into your lovemaking.

Men who can't ejaculate are frequently much too focused on their genitals. Sensate focus is a technique that was developed by Masters and Johnson to help couples get more in touch with all the sensations they are feeling. Sensate focus stresses the importance of touch and emphasizes building trust. When doing sensate focus, couples are encouraged to learn how to caress each other in a sensual way that doesn't necessarily lead to intercourse. (See page 223 for a sensate focus exercise that might improve your lovemaking.)

Don't give up too soon.

It took years for his DE to develop, so don't expect it to go away overnight. Don't be surprised if it takes several or, indeed, many attempts before he is able to masturbate to orgasm while you are present. What you need to measure is whether there is any difference in his ability to incorporate you into his sexual routine while he is masturbating. Does his capacity to make eye contact improve? Is he allowing your foreplay to become more sensual and intimate? If there is any change for the better, this is a good thing and signals the possibility that his DE could become a thing of the past. If these techniques fail the first or many times, don't immediately throw in the towel and assume a "nothing will work" attitude.

Put a time limit on your lovemaking sessions.

When I say don't give up, I don't mean to imply that you spend hours trying to force an ejaculation out of him. Find a loose time frame to which you both agree—let's say twenty to thirty minutes. You don't want to keep going so long that you end up feeling angry or resentful. Some men say that when having sex for a long time, they lose feeling in the penis or they know that they have gone beyond the point where an orgasm is possible. If this is true for him, ask him to tell you when he reaches that point because if his penis is no longer sensitive to what is going on, it's definitely time to stop.

See if he will agree to give up masturbating alone.

It's going to be very difficult to make headway if he continues to masturbate after you've made love. Remember, when he has an orgasm and ejaculates, it's a reflex. The more of an edge he has, the more likely it is that this reflex stands a chance of kicking in while the two of you are making love.

**Increase his comfort level by encouraging him to ejaculate
directly outside of your vagina.**

Some men become more comfortable with the idea of ejaculating
inside a vagina once they have been able to ejaculate near the vagina,
either directly outside or on the pubic area. Once he is able to ejaculate with you when he is masturbating, you can move on to doing
this. In fact, ejaculating anywhere on your body—between your
breasts or on your stomach—will help him become more comfortable
and help him get rid of some of his inhibitions about ejaculation.

Find creative ways to combine intercourse with masturbation.

Do these exercises once he is comfortable about masturbating in
front of you. They are also more likely to be successful if he has
been able to ejaculate by masturbating when you are with him. In
all of these exercises, he will be keeping his hands on his penis
while he is also thrusting into you. The following exercises combine intercourse with masturbation. When you are doing this, it
doesn't really matter if you start your lovemaking by masturbating
or with intercourse—whichever works best for you.

An exercise to try: This is an important exercise because it helps him
get over any reservations or inhibitions he might have about ejaculating during intercourse. Use the butterfly position and have him alternate thrusting into your vagina and masturbating. When he starts
coming with masturbation, have him thrust into your vagina. I've
used this exercise with clients with DE, and have had great results.

Another exercise: Masturbate together, with him lying on his
back. Once he says, "I'm coming" (and not a second before), jump
on top of him and finish up this way. The first few times you try

this technique, you may want to wait until semen actually starts to come out.

Other helpful positions: I have found that it sometimes helps if you get into positions that automatically tighten your vagina. Here are two examples:

1. Get into the missionary position. When he is on top of you, put one of your feet on top of the other and press down.

2. Get on your back. When he starts to thrust, raise your legs and spread them and use your hands to grab the arches of your feet.

THE GOOD NEWS: FOR MANY MEN, ONCE THEY HAVE MOVED PAST THEIR DIFFICULTY IN EJACULATING IN-SIDE A WOMAN AND HAVE BEEN ABLE TO DO IT ONCE OR TWICE, THE DE ISSUE JUST ABOUT DISAPPEARS.

5

He's Not Interested in Sex!

Susan met Jared six months ago, shortly after his divorce. Susan loves being with Jared; when they are together, she feels as though it is exactly where she belongs. He is very intense, very good-looking, and very smart. From her point of view, however, the relationship has a major problem. They don't have that much sex, and she doesn't know why. Jared is affectionate; he is romantic; almost every day he tells her how wonderful she is compared to his ex-wife, whom he describes as a cold woman who broke his heart when she slept with another guy. Susan's question is a simple one: "If he likes me so much, why doesn't he want to fool around?"

The first time Susan and Jared had sex, they were on their fourth date and had known each other two weeks. It was a Friday night, and Jared had a little bit too much to drink so the sex was far from memorable, but nonetheless Susan came away with the impression that Jared was a passionate guy who wanted her as much as she wanted him. Susan fell asleep that night curled up against Jared and looking forward to making love again the following morning or evening, or even sometime on Sunday—but it didn't happen. In fact, it was six dates and three more long weeks before Jared and Susan had sex again.

After a couple of months of dating, Susan figured out that three weeks is Jared's pattern. She has tried everything she could think of to get Jared in bed with greater frequency. She has maxed out her credit cards buying enticing clothing, shoes, and lingerie, and she has pressed her body against his in every way possible whenever she has had the chance. Short of tying him to the bed, Susan doesn't know what to do. Infrequent sex seems to suit Jared just fine. Susan, in the meantime, feels as though she is losing her mind. Jared is thirty-one, a young man. Susan, who is thirty-three, doesn't understand what is happening. Is it possible that Jared finds her too old? Does she need to lose weight? Wear shorter skirts and higher heels? Carry a whip? Use a stronger mouthwash? What is the problem? Her best friend told her that she should just confront Jared and ask him what is going on, and Susan wanted to do just that, but she never seemed to get the chance. The time was never right and the few times she tried to have this kind of conversation, Jared avoided the issue with the same kind of ease with which he has managed to avoid her physical overtures. What is the problem?

Embark on enough sexual relationships, and you will eventually find yourself with a man who wants to do only one thing in the bedroom—sleep. Perhaps no sexual issue is more emotionally distressing to a woman than being in a relationship with a guy who appears to be less passionate about her than she is about him. It can make her question everything about herself from the way she looks to the way she makes love. No matter what he tells her, or what she tells herself, the bottom line is that she frequently feels rejected. To further her unhappiness, she may find herself so consumed by unfulfilled desire that she can't think of anything else. Any woman who has ever fallen for a man who doesn't seem to be matching her in the passion department also knows that this situation creates a bizarre and unequal little power twist in the relationship; unwittingly, she becomes the pursuer and he becomes the adored love object. It feels pretty hideous.

If you find yourself in the unpleasant position of sharing a bed with a man who doesn't act like he wants to be there, the first thing you need to know is that in all likelihood, his lack of passion has nothing to do with you. It has nothing to do with whether you ate that last donut or whether your bathroom isn't spotless or whether your cat shredded his favorite shirt or your dog drooled on his new shoes. It also has nothing to do with the quality of your lingerie or the number of interesting positions into which you can arrange your body.

The other thing you need to know about low desire is that, for a man, it is a different issue from the inability to achieve an erection. In fact, a guy can have an erection with little or no desire to use it. Although limited desire is frequently named as the sexual issue of our times, there are a variety of reasons why it happens. Further, it usually means different things at different stages of your relationship. Finding out why your partner rarely wants sex is based on your current circumstances as well as history. Has this sexual pattern been present since the beginning of your relationship, for example? How old is your partner? What has recently changed in your relationship? Let's say your guy is thirty-two, and you've been dating for only a few months. Suddenly he stops initiating sex or starts avoiding it altogether. This is going to mean something very different from low sexual desire in the fifty-five-year-old guy who has been married to the same woman for twenty years.

If you consulted me as a sex therapist to talk about a man who doesn't appear to want to have sex, I would suggest that before you do anything else, you try to figure out the underlying reasons. Here are some questions to ask:

- Are there medical or physical reasons for his limited desire?
- Are problems in your relationship contributing to his issues with desire?
- Does he have an agenda (perhaps hidden) that includes avoiding sex with you?
- Does he have some serious psychological issues that translate into sexual behavior?

Let's look at these possibilities one by one.

THERE ARE MEDICAL OR PHYSICAL REASONS FOR HIS LIMITED DESIRE

Sometimes a man will complain that he is without desire or that his desire is very limited. If he has a long history of low desire, he may assume a lackadaisical attitude toward his limited libido. If, however, he is accustomed to thinking of himself as an insatiable guy, he may feel that his situation is very distressing. In fact, the guy whose sex drive is so low that it has fallen through the floorboards is often as distressed by his lack of libido as you are, perhaps more so. He may say that it takes so much to turn him on that it hardly seems worth the effort, and he may worry that there is something wrong with him, particularly if he thinks of himself as having a strong libido. During the course of a lifetime, just about every guy will go through stretches of time when his interest in sex is minimal. When this happens, it is usually because of one or a combination of the following reasons:

His testosterone levels have fallen.

This is rarely an issue when a man is in his twenties or thirties, but as he approaches his forties, fifties, and sixties, diminishing testosterone is definitely one of the factors connected to low desire and always needs to be taken into account. I have known men who had no difficulty having erections, but still lacked desire. This spells out low testosterone.

He has a medical problem.

If a man finds that his desire has all but disappeared, the best advice I can give is to tell him to schedule an appointment with his doctor. A wide variety of medical conditions such as diabetes, anemia, hypertension, or problems relating to the heart can make a guy lose his sexual oomph. Even a minor illness, such as a cold or flu, can interfere with sexuality. Exhaustion, which some men cite as a reason for their low libido, sometimes signals that there is an underlying medical issue.

He is depressed.

Depression is another common reason for a reduced interest in sex. Sometimes, life events such as the death of a loved one or serious work or money problems will topple a man into a depression without his even being fully aware of what's going on. People who suffer from depression typically say that when they are depressed they lose interest in everything, even activities as life-affirming as lovemaking. A man once told me, "I don't know if I am disinterested in sex because I'm depressed, or if I'm depressed because I'm not interested in sex."

He is taking one of many prescription medications that interfere with desire.

It would be difficult to list all the medications that disrupt sexual function. If you have a depressed lover, for example, the issue can be further complicated if he is taking an antidepressant medication that interferes with sexuality. Some of the most commonly prescribed are SSRIs (selective serotonin reuptake inhibitors) such as fluoxetine (Prozac), sertraline (Zoloft), or paroxetine (Paxil); these have all been cited as causing diminished libido as well as male erectile dysfunction. SNRIs (serotonin-norepinephrine reuptake inhibitors) such as venlafaxine (Effexor) can create similar reactions. Some of the medications used to treat ADD or ADHD can also bring sexual side effects. The same thing is true of some of the cholesterol-lowering medications. If he suffers from hypertension, his doctor may prescribe medication that affects sexuality. In short, any man who is taking any kind of medication and suffering from a low libido needs to have a serious conversation with his doctor *and* his pharmacist. An alternative medication may reverse the situation.

He's anxious or stressed.

There are some men who become so stressed by work or worry that it appears to block out all other feelings including desire. Sex is way down at the bottom of his priority list, someplace after finishing his taxes.

He has a problem with alcohol or drugs.

Some men can spend years abusing liquor or drugs without showing any sexual ill effects, but many others cannot. Low desire is but one of many sexual problems associated with drinking and drugs.

He's genuinely asexual.

It's estimated that 1.5 percent of the population are asexual. I've seen news stories recently talking about a group of such men and women who created a T-shirt that reads "Asexuality: It's not just for amoebas anymore." Those who describe themselves as asexual say that there is a distinction between celibacy, which is a choice, and asexuality, which is an asexual orientation. Many say that while they may want relationships and love, they don't feel desire and don't want sex.

PROBLEMS IN YOUR RELATIONSHIP ARE CONTRIBUTING TO HIS ISSUES WITH DESIRE

Contrary to popular belief, some men's sexual responses are deeply affected by the emotional interactions they have with their partners. They can sexually withdraw for any of the following reasons:

He is unhappy in the relationship.

Your relationship is going through a rocky phase, and he's not the kind of guy who is turned on by fighting. Maybe he's angry; maybe he's resentful, and the connection between the two of you is damaged. This doesn't necessarily mean that he wants to end the relationship, but it can mean that he is turned off and has surrounded himself with an almost impenetrable psychological wall.

He is bored by what is going on in your bedroom.

Boredom by itself will rarely be enough to stop a man from initiating sex, but let's say he has reached an age where he has diminished testosterone, is stressed at work, or absorbed by other things in his life, and the sex between the two of you has become routine at best. A guy like this can be much less interested in sex than he is in a Lakers game. If it's a new relationship, however, boredom is rarely going to be the reason for sexual disinterest.

He has some lazy sexual habits.

Some men just get into the habit of not having sex, and the less sex they have, the less sex they seem to need. A guy like this can be interested in a dozen other things, but sex with a woman seems like too much work and effort. It's easier to masturbate in the shower a couple of times a week. Sometimes when a man behaves this way, he and his sexual partner have a silent agreement that allows this situation to continue. He and his partner may have a great relationship, in which they agree about most things; they just don't have a very sexy relationship. He winks and says, "How about heading off to bed, sweetie?" She replies, "How about I bring you a beer and we watch another *Law & Order* rerun?" They both laugh and settle down in front of the TV. For the most part, sex takes a backseat to everything else.

HE HAS AN AGENDA (PERHAPS HIDDEN) THAT INCLUDES AVOIDING SEX WITH YOU

You need to understand that there is a distinction between the straightforward guy with minimal sex drive and the man who is avoiding sex. The avoider is usually very aware of what he is doing and presents a completely different scenario from somebody with genuinely low desire. The avoider typically has his reasons, which may include something that he is hiding. Over the years, I've heard many women complain about husbands and boyfriends who fall into this category. Typically, these women say things like, "I reach over for him in the middle of the night, and he rolls away from me." "He gets into bed at night and falls asleep (or pretends to fall asleep) before I get under the covers." "Whenever I try to hug him or kiss him, he moves away." "I feel certain that if we were to start anything, he would respond, but he avoids most body contact." "He tells me that it's not me, it's him, but why have we stopped making love?" Sometimes this behavior occurs suddenly in the middle of a long-term relationship; sometimes sexual avoidance is an issue from day one. Here are some common reasons.

He is seeing another woman (or women).

Yes, it is true that when your lover appears to be avoiding sex with you, he may well have a sexual attachment to someone else. My friend Deidre tells the story about the fiancé who called her at least five times a day to tell her how much he loved her. At night, however, he would avoid physical contact. Telling her that he adored her, he pleaded with her to please be patient. After three months of patience, she discovered that he was having prolonged lunch sex with a married woman in his office. It would be a mistake, however, to assume that all men who embark on new sexual relationships stop sleeping with their established partners. Many men can easily and seamlessly take on new partners without sexually disrupting the already-ongoing relationship.

He has a hidden outside sexual interest about which you are clueless.

I always remember the time my friend MaryLou met a smart, handsome, successful man who appeared to be very interested in her—so interested, in fact, that within weeks of their meeting, he invited her to move into his large, beautiful beach house. Everything was perfect, she thought, except that he didn't really want to have sex with her. After months of agonizing about what she could do to turn him on, MaryLou discovered the truth. Her "dream boyfriend" was only turned on by exceptionally tiny Asian women who were working in massage parlors. MaryLou is not the only woman to be unpleasantly surprised by a man's sexual inclinations. I once talked to a woman who discovered twenty years into the relationship that her accountant husband was spending four nights a week at an S&M club. When he went out, he usually told her that he was either going to the library to study for a graduate degree or to choir practice. Here's how she found out the truth: She was vacuuming and when she pushed his bureau away from the wall, she found several snapshots of him, naked on his hands and knees wearing a dog collar. Standing over him was a towering blonde holding a whip.

He really prefers men.

More than one woman has cried herself to sleep at night after learning that the reason the man in her life didn't want to have sex with her was because he didn't really want to have sex with *any* woman. My friend Gretchen was married to her husband Phil for fifteen years. He was never the most passionate lover in the world, but they managed to have two children. She complained that with every year of their marriage, he became more creative about finding excuses for not having sex. She was a normal woman, and at first she followed all the advice she read in *Cosmo* about massage oils and whipped cream. After a while she became too embarrassed and humiliated by what was going on, so she gave up. To the outside world, their marriage looked reasonably normal, and they were good friends. Finally, one day he confessed that he was "living a lie" and couldn't continue one day longer. He was gay! In retrospect, she says that she should have figured it out—but at the time, she claims she had no idea, and I believe her.

He is insecure about his skills as a lover or overwhelmed by performance pressure.

This is most likely to happen when the guy either is very young and inexperienced or over forty-five and beginning to notice a decline in testosterone. Young men can sexually withdraw because they don't really know what to do, or worry that they won't measure up. They may worry about penis size, getting an erection, whether they will ejaculate too soon, and whether or not they can please a woman. Older men, who are less capable of having and maintaining erections than they once were, sometimes start avoiding sex because they think they just can't do it effectively anymore.

He discovered that he has an STD and doesn't know how to tell you.

You just met the most attractive guy at the gym. He asks you out. You go to the movies and out to dinner. He avoids physical contact. Six weeks later, you're still going out, and he still hasn't touched you. He has sort of implied that there is something he has to tell you. You worry he will confess that he's wanted for homicide in Montana and start googling for information about *America's Most Wanted*. This kind of behavior can also happen with a man you've known for a while: In that case, he starts looking for excuses not to have sex or begins whipping out condoms like they are going out of style.

He thinks he is still in love with another woman.

Typically this is a woman from his past—an ex-wife or girlfriend. Your relationship may start off with what appears to be a great deal of sexual promise, but it fizzles rapidly, and you don't know why. Because he likes you (and because he's the kind of guy who is lost without an ongoing relationship), he continues to date you. If he were to try to explain his behavior to you or a friend, he probably wouldn't be able to do so. He might tell himself that he is hoping eventually he will forget about the ex-love. I've met variations of this guy who were more than willing to have intercourse with a new woman, but drew the line at kissing or much affection. Obviously, they were also a little bit nuts.

He's uptight about sex.

Something in his personal background or belief system has made him repressed about anything sexual, and he may not want that to change. For example, I had a friend once who started to date a very religious guy. He was in his early thirties; he had never had sex; and he was reluctant to have sex until he was married. They decided to get married, but she was so turned on and anxious to get him into bed that they had a secret marriage six months before their scheduled wedding date. Within weeks, she was complaining that he wasn't interested in having sex. Well, duh! If a guy has reached the age of thirty without ever having sex, that's kind of a tip-off. Men who are uptight about sex usually let you know about it in dozens of ways, large and small.

He's angry at you, and he's trying to get even.

It does happen, honest. Perhaps he thinks you have done something that is unforgivable like accidentally front-ending his car or sleeping with his best friend; or perhaps he is harboring years of anger. Whatever the reason, this guy has figured out that sex is important to you. So why not hold out?

He's more interested in Internet porn than he is in a real relationship.

This was certainly never an issue when I first started seeing clients, but it has become more and more prevalent in the last ten years. Jill, for example, is very upset because her new boyfriend Ben rarely sleeps over. When they have sex, it's terrific, but he only wants sex every ten days or so. They've only been dating for a few months. In all her previous relationships, the early stages were marked by nonstop sex and long weekends in bed. Ben has shown no interest in this kind of activity. When Ben leaves Jill at night and goes home, she often turns on her computer to answer e-mails. When Ben gets home, she can see that he gets online also. With a little bit of Internet sleuthing on her part, she has managed to figure out that he is online every night until the wee small hours of the morning. She asked him what was going on, and he acknowledged that he loves Internet porn. He thinks that this behavior of his is perfectly normal, and he doesn't want to change it. She thinks that she needs a guy who wants to spend more time in her bed.

He has taken a vow of celibacy.

He may be a very sexy guy, but for reasons many of us can't begin to comprehend, he believes that celibacy is part of his spiritual journey. He may vow to remain celibate only until he marries, or he may be committed to living as a monk for years or even for the rest of his life. There is also another bizarre twist to contemporary celibacy vows. There are men who genuinely believe that as far as sexual celibacy is concerned, the only thing that counts is intercourse and that they have a free pass on all other sexual activities. From my point of view, the best thing about the guy who has taken a vow of celibacy is that he usually tells you about it.

He's avoiding commitment; he doesn't want to let it become more intimate.

Remember Susan, who I talked about at the beginning of this chapter, and how she wanted to know why Jared had so little interest in sex? Well, after about six months of dating, Jared finally broke up with Susan. He told her that he realized that she wanted more from a relationship than he wanted to give. It was too soon after his divorce and he wasn't ready for a commitment. Susan asked him about the sex. He told her that he had purposely been limiting the sex in order to make sure that the relationship didn't move forward too quickly.

I know this sounds stupid, but some men honestly believe that if they are able to limit the amount of sex in a relationship, they will be able to put a brake on the relationship. Their reasoning goes something like this: In a committed relationship, you can have sex whenever you want it, so if we only have sex every couple of weeks or so, it means that this is still a casual dating relationship. In their heads, sex and commitment go together, just like love and marriage. If the relationship breaks up and the woman complains, he might think something along the lines of "She had to know it wasn't serious. After all, we only had sex every ten days."

HE HAS SOME SERIOUS PSYCHOLOGICAL ISSUES

Thirty years ago, it was generally assumed that the majority of sexual issues were psychological, and physiology was given short shrift.

Back then, if a man began to experience sexual difficulties and talked to his doctor about his complaints, no matter what the underlying cause, he would almost inevitably be told to discuss his issues with a psychiatrist. Today, things have changed and we can all be grateful for it. Nonetheless, when a woman is having a relationship with a man who doesn't appear to want sex, she needs to consider the possibility that psychological factors may be involved. These include:

He has Madonna/whore issues.

Penny met Hugh at a friend's wedding. From the moment they met, his M.O. was hot pursuit. On the second date, he began to talk about moving in together, getting married, and having children. Hugh mowed Penny down with his passion and intensity; she says she began to fall in love with him simply because he liked her so much. It was wonderful being with a man who acted as though he adored her. The first few times they had sex, it was pretty good. They had known each other less than three months when Hugh proposed, convincing Penny to give up her apartment and move in with him. From the day she and her cat arrived, the sex changed. It became almost nonexistent. Penny thought that perhaps Hugh was having prewedding jitters and that things would improve after the wedding. Well, in fact, after the wedding, the sexual relationship didn't improve. If anything, it got worse. They have been married almost a year and Penny feels cheated by the lack of sex. She knows Hugh needs sex because she can't ignore his middle of the night and morning erections; from the noises in the shower each morning, she suspects that he is masturbating with a fair amount of regularity. What is Hugh's agenda?

Here and now in the twenty-first century, it almost seems like a joke to talk about something that sounds as archaic as a Madonna/whore complex. In this post-Freudian world, haven't men outgrown that kind of thing? I wish this were the case, but the sad truth is that there are definitely men who can't seem to handle sex within the context of a committed relationship. They separate women into two categories—"good" girls who they marry and "bad" girls who they save for sex. By the way, if you should meet one of these men, the category into which he places you frequently has nothing to do with the reality of the situation. You could be the sexiest woman who ever lived, but if something about you fits into his preconceived ideas about wife and mother, that's where he will fit you in. Conversely, you could be a white-gloved Sunday school teacher, and if he finds you incredibly appealing, in his head you could become the woman who was meant for sex and sex alone. Although it's true that some men like this are most comfortable having sex with professionals, it would be a mistake to think in terms of stereotypes. Remember that his response to women and sex is originating in his head.

If you should meet a guy like this and he sees you as the "good girl" who was meant for a committed relationship, he will typically either not have sex with you or only have sex with you infrequently, preferring to leave you on your sex-starved pedestal. If he sees you as the sex symbol, it will be almost impossible for him ever to regard you as "wife and mother material." Getting involved with this guy is clearly a no-win situation.

He suffers from sexual aversion disorder.

There is a huge difference between a man with low desire who doesn't want to have sex and a man who is actually phobic at the idea of sex. He could be afraid of everything about sex, or he could have a specific phobia such as the fear of being touched or fear of going down on a woman. The person with a sexual aversion disorder frequently has the phobic symptoms to prove it—rapid heartbeat, diarrhea, sweating, or nausea. Masters and Johnson, who treated a fair number of people with sexual aversion issues, said that the primary causes are: "(1) Severely negative parental sex attitudes; (2) a history of sexual trauma (e.g., rape, incest); (3) a pattern of constant sexual pressuring by a partner in a long-term relationship; and (4) gender identity confusion in men." Further, they said that their success rate in treating sexual aversion was over 80 percent even in cases of long duration.

He's addicted to masturbation.

I am a huge proponent of masturbation, but not at the expense of the sexuality that exists between two people. If he is so happy satisfying himself that there is no place in his bed for a woman, he may have an autoerotic psychological orientation. If so, he is *very* unlikely to change.

QUESTIONS TO ASK YOURSELF

If you find yourself sharing a bed with a man who appears to have limited desire, I'm not going to tell you to rush out immediately and buy some new lingerie or learn some new fancy sexual tricks. Instead, I'm going to ask you to evaluate the situation realistically.

You have to start by getting answers to three huge relationship questions:

Is he prepared to work with you on the issue of his low desire? If he doesn't take your concerns seriously or acts as if you are nagging him, then let's face it, there is very little that you can do to fix things.

Are you prepared to find out why he doesn't want sex as much as you do? This could be a tough situation. You may be worried that he is seeing another woman (or man) or you may be worried that he is backing away from the relationship. I personally always believe in getting as many facts out in the open as possible, but I understand what it is to be nervous about discovering something that could completely change or disrupt your life.

Is it possible that you are also more comfortable in a relationship in which there is little sex? Some women also get lazy about sex. They may be exhausted from jobs and children and a variety of daily demands. They may begin to think things like "Well, one good thing about not having sex is that I don't have to shave my legs as often." In an earlier era, these are the women who headed off to bed wearing curlers and face cream. Today, these are the women who at eleven P.M. can sometimes be found wearing their teenage son's flannel "jammies," polishing off a pint of Ben & Jerry's, doing a load of laundry, and watching *Sex and the City* reruns.

HE'S NOT INTERESTED IN SEX: WHAT CAN YOU DO?

Although you are absolutely not responsible for his low desire, there are still things that you can and should do.

1. Ask him to consult with a medical professional for a complete medical checkup. I cannot stress enough how important it is to rule out any potential underlying medical conditions, whether they be physical or psychological.

2. If medical issues have been ruled out, talk with him honestly. You need to know if there are problems in the relationship that can be resolved. You also need to know if the situation is hopeless.

3. *See a therapist together.* Is he willing to go with you to talk to a therapist or counselor? Perhaps in the context of a counselor's office, he might be more forthcoming about what he thinks is going awry with his libido. A therapist might have some simple concrete suggestions that could help.

4. *If one of the issues between you as a couple is stress or boredom, you need to find ways to reconnect as a couple.* When a couple has been together for more than a few years, they absolutely do fall into romantic ruts. Frequently, this is incredibly easy to resolve. A vacation, a few romantic dinners, and a change of scenery can work wonders. Try to remember what it is that he finds exciting and try to connect with him around it. If he loves baseball, for example, go with him to root for his favorite team. Enthusiasm and passion will often carry over into the sexual arena. Try to find new ways to approach each other sexually. (Check out the sensate focus exercise on page 223.)

5. *See a therapist separately for yourself.* If you come to the conclusion that your partner is avoiding sex or avoiding you, you may need professional help in order to deal with the issues in your relationship appropriately and realistically. A couple of things can happen to a woman who is in this kind of a situation: She may inappropriately blame herself for what isn't happening in her bedroom, or she may start feeling generally undesirable. This is one of those times in life when it's good to have the support of others to help you understand what is happening. You may, for example, decide that you want to end your relationship, and you may need some support in doing this. If you can't financially afford an individual therapist, perhaps there is some kind of support group that

you can join. Co-Dependents Anonymous, for example, states that the only requirement for membership "is a desire for healthy and loving relationships."

6. *Take care of yourself.* I know that you are a sexual woman. Otherwise you wouldn't be reading this book. I also know how easy it is for a woman's ego to get beaten down when she is in a relationship with a reluctant lover or a man whose behavior is making her feel less than desirable. Right now, you need to do things that make you feel attractive and sensual. This is where you get to buy new underwear, but don't do it to turn your partner on. Do it in order to pamper yourself. Join a gym, get a pedicure. Do whatever you can to help you feel like the sexual, desirable woman you are.

The main thing is for you to make sure your own libido doesn't suffer just because he isn't interested. You owe it to yourself to find someone who is. Make sure you keep up with self-touch, erotic literature or movies, and sensual experiences like spa treatments and long, luxurious baths. Also make sure that you stay physically fit, because it's a huge boost for your libido and sense of self.

6

Do You Like What He Likes?

Back in Grandma and Great-Grandma's day, if people talked about sex, which of course they never did, you could pretty much assume they were talking about intercourse. That's because of the common belief that until the sexual revolution, intercourse, usually done silently and in the missionary position, was the primary activity going on in the bedrooms of America. Nowadays, of course, most of us have been exposed to information (not to mention photographs) concerning people doing just about everything and in every position imaginable, and not always in the privacy of their bedrooms, either. Let's acknowledge it: We live in a sexually experimental society. This is something I love, but not all of you may feel the same way. Even if I disagree with you, however, I respect and honor your right to be as sexually loose or conservative as you want to be. Your sexual comfort zone is something you have to establish for yourself.

When you begin a sexual relationship with a man, you and he are going to have to decide together what kinds of things you want to do, and how you want to do them. I'm not talking here about group sex, or S&M, or sex in public places. I'm talking about fairly run-of-the-mill sexual practices that a fair number of your neighbors and friends have also tried. Nonetheless there are some sexual practices that men may or may not like, and that some women may like more than others.

ORAL SEX

I'm sure someplace in this great constellation we all inhabit, there is a man who doesn't like having a woman perform oral sex on him. However, I have never met this man, nor do I know any other woman who has met him. I've never even heard stories along the lines of "I have a friend, who has a friend, who once met this guy who claimed that he didn't like oral sex until he met her."

The formal word for performing oral sex on a man is *fellatio*. (When a guy is performing oral sex on you, it's called *cunnilingus*.) It wasn't that long ago that oral sex was considered a particularly risqué practice. That's all changed. Nowadays, everybody seems to be doing it. One of the big issues with oral sex is that some people don't consider it sex. Many teenagers, for example, along with some well-known politicians, fall into this category.

Since I have noticed nighttime cable shows giving very explicit how-to advice on how to perform oral sex, I'm sure you know what needs to be done. You can practice using a spoon, a Popsicle, a large lollipop, or even a dildo. All you need to do is keep warm, wet pressure on a man's penis while you move your head up and down. If you do that, you've got great odds that nature will take its course. In other words, there are no hard and fast rules as to how to perform oral sex. It comes down to a matter of how you feel and how you enjoy doing it. Here are some suggestions to help you enjoy it more.

1. Make sure you are comfortable when you start. There is nothing worse than getting into an awkward position while a guy is getting more and more excited. I've been there so I know what happens then. You don't want to interrupt the guy or ruin his erection or orgasm by stopping what you are doing, but you also know that if you continue much longer, you're going to be spending the next week with a stiff neck. It's important that you take the time to find a position in which you are able to relax. You might want to kneel in front of your partner. You might want to sit in a chair while he stands. You might want to lie on your side on a bed while he kneels on the bed. If he is lying on his back, you can kneel over him. If he is lying on his side on the bed, you can lie next to him with a pillow under your neck.

2. You can control how much or how little of your partner's penis is going into your mouth if you keep your hand around the base of his penis so you are in charge of the depth of penetration. This is particularly important if you are worried about gagging.

3. With oral sex, remember that you are in charge and the man is the more passive partner. In intercourse (particularly if he is on top or even on the side), men tend to control the movement. With oral sex, you set the pacing, and you control the movement. It's all about how fast or slow you want to move. Ask him how he likes it, but don't be afraid to experiment and tease him a bit.

4. Don't be afraid to use both your hand and your mouth. You can use your hand to stroke back and forth on the penis, much as a man might do if he were masturbating, while your mouth focuses on the head of the penis and directly beneath it. Again, this is a way of making sure you are less likely to gag from depth of penetration.

5. Don't forget his testicles. When you start, you can gently suck on his testicles, one at a time. Don't forget to lick the area right

behind the testicles. While you are using your mouth to perform oral sex on his penis, he might like it if you keep one hand on his penis while the other one focuses on his testicles.

6. Don't be nervous about asking him where he wants you to place your hands and how much pressure he wants you to apply. Ask him to use his own hands to show you. Trust me, it's very sexy. It's also a good way to help him get over his inhibitions.

7. When performing oral sex, remember that enthusiasm is the most important ingredient. He is more turned on when you are turned on.

8. I know you don't need me to tell you to keep your lips around your teeth so that you don't end up biting him. I never actually heard of a guy being bitten during oral sex, but some men worry about the possibility, at least a little bit.

9. Use a lot of tongue, and always keep everything wet—very wet.

10. Remember that oral sex is no protection against STDs.

MEN AND PORNOGRAPHY

There have always been naked bodies, and almost as soon as cameras were invented, people started taking pictures of them. But is that pornography? What is pornography anyway? A famous, often-quoted statement about pornography comes from a legal opinion by a Supreme Court justice who basically said that he couldn't define it, and then continued on to say, "But I know it when I see it . . ."

In this country, pornography as big business probably started back in 1953, when Hugh Hefner founded *Playboy* magazine; the very first edition of the magazine (filled with pictures of a young, unknown, and unclothed Marilyn Monroe) was published without a date because Hefner wasn't sure it would be around long enough for there to be another edition. (When someone later asked Monroe about the photo shoot, she said in that whispery voice of hers, "It's not true I had nothing on. I had the radio on.") It goes without saying that the magazine sold out almost immediately, and the rest is history. Back then, many considered *Playboy* to be the last word in pornography. When we look back at those old *Playboy*s, they seem almost innocent compared to the kind of porn that is currently available, some of it even packaged as art. Recently, a new drama debuted on HBO filled with some pretty graphic sex scenes. One of the scenes featured a young couple making love. The camera shot gave the viewer a really extraordinary look at the guy's balls. I might not remember the actor's face, but I think I would recognize those balls anywhere. The question is, do shots like these turn women on? Many women would answer, "No!" But show a similarly intimate shot of a woman's backside or breasts and ask whether men would be excited, and the answer would probably be "Hell, yes!"

A distinction is often made between hard-core and soft-core porn. Traditionally, the difference was that soft-core did not show male full frontal nudity, erections, or penetration. Hard-core, of course, would show all of these. These distinctions have become blurred because of pressure from the cable sex networks, so the hard-core/soft-core distinction does not apply in some domains. Rather, they are trying to make a distinction of violent versus nonviolent, or showing consenting adults versus non.

When it comes to porn, men and women may have different reactions. Studies have been done that show that both men and women are physically turned on by sexually explicit material. The difference is that men usually recognize and acknowledge that they are excited and are prepared to act on that excitement. Women, on the other hand, have a different reaction. Even if they are physically aroused, their arousal may lack the psychological component they need in order to take the next step and have sex. A woman, for example, might be lubricating, but if her emotional reaction is that she finds what she is viewing offensive, she is more likely to say, "Gross. I don't want to do that!"

It would almost appear that most women have a built-in censor that keeps them from acting on their strictly physical sexual reactions, but who knows—that may all change with another generation.

Two of the most common questions women ask about porn are:

He's very interested in pornography. Is there something wrong with him? The answer to that depends at least in part on the kind of porn. If he is fascinated, for example, by kiddie porn, I might question his fascination as well as his viability for a relationship. I might also have some serious concerns if he is primarily interested in porn that is cruel or violent or has strong misogynistic themes. I would also want to know how much time he spends watching porn. If he is consistently more interested in watching porn than he is in making love with a partner, this does not bode well for his capacity to have a sexual relationship. If he is in a heterosexual relationship with you, but the porn that he chooses to watch is primarily gay, then I would also wonder whether he is being honest about his sexual orientation.

But if the guy in your life has an interest and curiosity in viewing explicitly sexual material that for the most part features passionate straight couples, I would tend to think that he is just a normal guy with a normal interest. (I might also add here that many average guys also fantasize about the idea of viewing women having sex with each other.) In short, just because he has an interest in porn (as opposed to an obsession) doesn't mean that he's weird or going to turn weirder.

He's very interested in porn. Does that mean that there's something wrong with me? Some women worry that their partner's interest in porn means that something is wrong with him, but just as many women worry that it means that there is something wrong with them. Take Bonnie, for example. She says, "When I met him, my husband had a small stack of pornographic videos and magazines. Now he has a good-size stack of DVDs. He keeps them in the back of his bedroom closet so the children can't find them. At least a couple of nights a month, he goes into the den and watches them when he thinks I'm asleep and not going to notice. He says it is harmless and it relaxes him. I wish I wasn't disturbed by this, but I am. When he looks at all these incredible-looking women with those amazing bodies—even if their boobs aren't real—I can't help but feel that I'm getting failing grades in the looks department. These women he looks at make me feel fat and dumpy and boring-looking. I'm ashamed to admit it, but they make me jealous. If this is what he wants, I don't know why he married me. Yes, it's true I knew before we got married that he sometimes watched porn, but I guess I thought he was going to outgrow it, or once we were together all the time and he could have sex whenever he wanted it, he would lose interest in porn. If anything, he seems more interested."

I think it's important for Bonnie and women like her to relax and stop feeling threatened just because a guy watches a little bit of porn. For the most part, it absolutely does not mean that he finds his sexual partner any less attractive; it absolutely does not mean that he loves her less. All it means is that he is a guy who has a small porn habit, which may stimulate his sexual fantasy life.

When a guy watches a great deal of porn, however, it can alter the way he looks at sex in his own relationship. Some research now indicates that when men watch a lot of porn, they become dissatisfied with their own bodies, their own sexual performance, their partners' bodies, and their partners' sexual performance. This is kind of an insidious effect because all of the porn actors and actresses are so spectacularly good-looking compared to the almost average-looking players who were involved in the porn industry back in the 1970s.

There are other issues that can be connected to the regular viewing of pornography. Suppose a guy, let's call him Jim, starts out watching some soft porn, which he finds exciting, but after viewing material like this for a while, he graduates to porn that is a little edgier. After a few weeks, months, or even years, Jim no longer finds this level stimulating, so he starts looking for material that is even more hard-core. Eventually Jim might possibly become a porn addict who might find himself more interested in watching porn than he is in canoodling with his significant other. As I've said before, the biggest problem with porn is if the man becomes compulsive or starts preferring porn to sex. This behavior indicates a more serious issue that needs to be addressed and may require some counseling. (We go into this more in the next chapter.)

Many women enjoy watching soft porn with their partners because it can be a terrific turn-on. I always advise couples who want to incorporate porn into their lovemaking that they should watch "just enough" porn. By "just enough" I mean watching enough porn to increase desire and boost the number of times they want to have sex, but not so much that they become jaded and need more and more stimulation and hard-core stuff to get turned on.

While I'm one of those women who enjoys some soft-core porn, I'm also aware that sex between two people is an intimate and sensitive act. I think it can be a real mistake to desensitize yourself to the point where you need to view wilder and wilder stimulation. I also think it's a mistake to believe that sex has to be the way it is on the screen in order to be interesting. For me, sincere, sensitive sex is more enticing than performance sex.

SEX TOYS

There are, of course, a wide variety of sex toys sold, but the ones most commonly used in heterosexual relationships are vibrators and dildos. And yes, it is absolutely true that women are the biggest purchasers of this kind of sex toy. Men still tend to be the primary purchasers of porn DVDs, but apparently, the number of women buying them has greatly increased. I think men are still more likely to be the ones buying bondage apparatus. This can range from novelty items such as mink handcuffs with Velcro closures or satin blindfolds to the more serious equipment such as whips and chains. So if you are in bed with a man and he brings out the mink handcuffs, there is probably no cause for concern. If he starts pulling out serious bondage gear, run! Unless, of course, you're into that.

A few years back, women often felt that guys were threatened by vibrators. I don't think that's true any longer. In fact, most men like to use them. After all, is there anything a guy likes more than expensive equipment or gear? He buys it for biking, sailing, or mountain climbing—why not for sex? A guy's solution to learning a new skill or sport is always to buy a bunch of expensive equipment. With sex, however, you often have to be the one to teach a man how to use a vibrator or dildo on you. Men can be too enthusiastic or heavy-handed. You want to stress that you are using a dildo or vibrator for sensuality, not as a pile driver or Makita drill. If a man thinks you like sex toys, you run the risk that he's going to go down to Condom Revolution and buy out the store. Make sure he knows that you are the one who needs to pick them out. I've been on the receiving end of new sex toys (literally) too many times. Guys have shown up at my house with the strangest things. The worst was this cock ring thing with nubs on it that were supposed to stimulate your clitoris. I was sore for three days. Never again!

FANTASIES IN YOUR BEDROOM

Incorporating fantasy into your lovemaking can be fun; it can be frightening; it can be intimidating; it can be infuriating; or it can be exciting and arousing. It depends upon several things including:

Your attitude toward sex and lovemaking

Let's say you are a romantic, relatively inexperienced woman. The chances are that you are going to be totally turned off by fantasies that offend your romantic sensibility. You want sex to be between you and the man you love. Any sense that you are being asked to pretend that he is somebody else or you are somebody else may be offensive. On the other hand, you might find yourself aroused by fantasies that incorporate your romantic nature and increase the level of intimacy between you and your partner. Some women, of course, are experimental by nature and they love sex that crosses the line. If you are one of these women, you might get a real kick out of some wilder fantasies.

The kind of fantasies he enjoys

There are a wide variety of different kinds of fantasies and over the years, I have heard women talk about some of the things their partners suggested and how they suggested it. For example, Ellie says that her fiancé brought home some exquisite lingerie for her and told her that he wanted to see her in it because she was so beautiful. He said he thought it would be fun to pretend that she was a lovely sleeping princess and he was a visitor who couldn't contain himself and brought her to life with oral sex. She said that it ended up being a total turn-on. On the other hand, Betty Anne says that when they had sex, her ex-husband wanted her to pretend that she was having sex with someone else and tell him about it. She went along with his requests, but she hated it. As far as she was concerned her husband's fantasies had nothing to do with intimacy and caused her to distance herself from him and the relationship. She says her husband's fantasies turned sex into something she endured as opposed to enjoyed.

Of course, some couples are meant for each other. He loves acting out the role of submissive love slave; she adores talking to him as though he is a meaningless, worthless crumb on the bedroom floor. Or perhaps they both believe they were pirates in an earlier life and derive pleasure from screaming, "Ahoy matey!" to each other when they have orgasms. Hey, whatever works. All we can do is envy these couples.

His attitude toward you and how this is reflected in his fantasies

For the most part, women love fantasies that make them feel special and adored and connected. They tend to dislike fantasies that make them feel alienated, alone, and depersonalized by their partners. They don't like scenarios in which they feel as though they are being forced to cater to what appears to them to be some creepy guy's even creepier inner life.

If you and your partner are going to use fantasy in your bedroom, you really have to know yourself and the two of you have to work it out very carefully. If he is indulging in fantasies that feel destructive, and you go along with it, it can feel almost as though you are under attack. This morning on the television, there was a news report about a woman who shot her preacher husband. One of the reasons cited is that he was asking her to wear a wig and platform heels to excite him. She felt abused by his requests. This is probably an understatement, but it would have definitely been better if she had been able to talk about it.

How often he brings his fantasies into your lovemaking

The other issue to consider is how often your partner wants to include fantasy in your sex life. Perhaps you enjoy a little fantasy every now and again, but you prefer sex to feel more intimate and connected. On the other hand, perhaps you adore having sex with an element of let's pretend, and your partner doesn't. These are the issues that a couple needs to negotiate.

Are your bedroom fantasies making anyone jealous?

Some women ask me, "Will sharing fantasies with my partner bring us closer?" I usually advise against you and your partner sharing fantasies that involve another person unless you both are in the very small percentage of the population who have no sexual jealousy whatsoever. What if he tells you he has been fantasizing about having sex with your sister? Or your mother? Or your best friend?

How are you going to react? How will he react if you tell him you fantasize about somebody else?

Some advice about fantasies

My final word when it comes to fantasies is that a couple should talk them through carefully before they are having sex. Remember, sex is something that is happening between two people. You can't be having good sex if one partner's head is off in an S&M dungeon while the other wants no part of it.

ANAL SEX

"Come on honey, let's try it. I promise I'll be gentle and I promise I'll stop the minute you tell me to stop. Please."

In bedrooms across America, men are uttering words like this to their often-reluctant partners. Of course, what they are talking about is anal sex.

Before reading further, let me tell you a little story, which may or may not have anything to do with anal sex. I have this girl-friend I've known since we were teenagers. She has been happily married to her first real boyfriend in a monogamous relationship since she was in her early twenties; she is as sexually conservative as I am experimental. She has a really great disposition and fabulous, loud laugh, and I often wait to tell her jokes until we are in public, just so she'll laugh and make everybody turn around. Once we were near a ski resort in Colorado, and I asked her if she had ever been skiing, and she said yes, which surprised me because I don't think of her as being athletic. She asked me if I had ever been skiing, and I said, "No, to me skiing is like anal sex, I don't have to do it to know I wouldn't like it." So we were walking into a store, and she said, "So, have you ever done it?" And I said, "Skiing? No way!" And of course she started whooping with laughter, which caused everybody in the whole town to turn around to look at her.

The idea of anal sex always seems to make some people laugh. Even so, statistically, the number of heterosexual men and women who are indulging in it is growing. At least 25 percent have tried it at least once in their lives and about 5 to 10 percent do it regularly—and these numbers would appear to be on an upswing. I also want to make it clear right here that anal sex is not just about anal intercourse. It includes a whole range of anal sex play from fingers, licking, inserting objects such as dildos, scarves, and Ben Wa balls, all the way to anal intercourse.

I don't know why so many men are so gung ho about the idea of anal sex, but if you go to bed with more than a few guys, statistically you are probably going to meet one who is determined to get you to indulge him on this level. Women tend to be much less experimental about this and many quickly dismiss the idea of trying it, saying words along the lines of "Ychhhh!!! No way!!!" There are other women, however, who are totally into anal sex. Many say that combined with clitoral or vaginal stimulation, anal penetration provides stupendous orgasms. One woman I know told me that under the right conditions and with the right person, she absolutely loves anal sex. What she particularly enjoys is having a man use his fingers to penetrate her anus. She says that she has had several incredible orgasms this way that she would describe as "whole body experiences."

If you are completely opposed to the idea of anal sex, just say no! You don't have to do it, and it does not have to be part of your bedroom repertoire. Some wise guy once said something along the lines of "Women will usually go along with anal sex twice. The first time to see what it feels like, and the second time to make sure that it was really as painful as she thought it was." Many women say that they agreed to try anal sex, not because they wanted to try it but because they really wanted to please their partners. They say they are so much in love, or so sexually excited and passionate about their significant others, that they want to do whatever it is he wants to do. I'm not sure this kind of thinking always presents the wisest motivation in the world.

If you do decide you want to have anal sex with a guy, here are some things you need to know.

- Make sure you are relaxed. When you are tense, the whole body tightens up, including the anus. To have any kind of anal penetration, you need to be relaxed and comfortable.
- Use lots and lots of lubrication. I mean lots!
- It's wisest if you don't start out by letting him insert his penis. Start slowly with his fingers. Start with one, see how it feels. Graduate to two, then three. Don't go for penile insertion until you know you are relaxed and comfortable with what is taking place. It may take several sessions of lovemaking before you are ready to progress to actual penile insertion.
- It's going to be a lot better for you if the guy you are with knows what he is doing. Ask him to read up on the subject. There are actually books written about it. One that is particularly good is *Anal Pleasure & Health*. It's written by a sex therapist named Jack Morin. If you and your partner want to try anal sex, this is something you should both read. In my experience, a funny thing happens when people read Jack Morin's book. The men, who initially were all gung ho, often decide not to do it, because they didn't realize it was going to

be this much trouble. The women, who were initially reluctant, often begin to think, hey, this is something that a lot of people do, and it might not be that bad. In fact, with the right preparation, it might be okay.

- Recognize the risks of anal sex. Unless you and your partner are careful, you do run the risk of causing cuts and tears as well as other physical damage to the rectum and anus, which can require medical treatment.

There is a risk of spreading HIV and HPV, as well as other STDs, with anal penetration. This is because there are likely to be small fissures and tears in the anus. That's why it's best to use a condom. Also, there is a greater likelihood of a condom tearing during anal sex than during vaginal sex.

There is a real risk of spreading bacteria from the anus to the vagina or the urethra. This can result in a urinary tract infection. If that's not bad enough, in some instances this can lead to a kidney infection. If you are going to have anal sex, you and your partner need to be careful. It's not a good idea to insert an object into the vagina that has been in the anus without washing it; it doesn't matter whether that object is a sex toy, a finger, or a penis. It needs to be carefully cleansed.

A FINAL WORD OF WARNING

Do not, I repeat, do not allow your partner to put anything up your butt and do not put anything up his unless there is a handle or some other secure way of removing it. There are too many horror stories about people ending up in emergency rooms. The story about the woman going to the ER with a Pocket Rocket in her rectum still vibrating is not just another urban myth. It can happen. One of the other things I always tell clients and students is that a penis should never be put into a vacuum cleaner. Inevitably somebody will then ask me, "Well, who would do that?" I always have the same answer, which is, "You'd be surprised."

7

Is There Such a Thing as a Sex Addict? Could He Be One of Them?

After four years of marriage, Marnie is thinking of leaving her husband, Todd. When she first met him and they spent hours (and sometimes days) in bed, she loved it. She loved having sex, and she loved that he was such a hot guy. He told her that whenever she walked into the room he got an erection. It was exciting to be with somebody who made her feel so desirable. Now, however, she is ready to scream, "Enough already!" Todd expects to have sex every single morning and every single night as well as dozens of other times in between. Marnie says that they can't go anywhere without first having sex. As an example, when Marnie's mother was hospitalized for emergency surgery, Todd insisted on having sex before Marnie rushed to the hospital. A day later, while a worried Marnie sat at her sleeping mother's hospital bedside, Todd showed up to visit. At first Marnie was really glad to see him, but when he suggested that they find an empty supply closet in which they could have sex, all Marnie wanted was for him to go away. Todd's preoccupation with sex has turned Marnie off. She says, "He's always after me, and I've figured out that it has very little to do with me. I hate it."

Phoebe is getting more and more fed up with Dave, the guy she lives with. When Phoebe first met Dave, he was recently divorced.

When he told Phoebe how much his wife nagged him, Phoebe promised him that she would never turn into a nag. Now, Phoebe is beginning to have a greater understanding of his ex-wife's point of view. When Dave and Phoebe first started going out, she got the impression that he wasn't that interested in sex. She thought he was a guy with a low sex drive, which she was prepared to tolerate because of other good things in the relationship. Now that they are living together, and she sees what he does every night, she says, "It's not that he isn't interested in sex. It's that he's not interested in sex with me, or with anyone else who is human. All he's interested in is the sex that's going on every night on his computer screen. After I go to bed, that's what he does, late into the night. I have no idea what kind of porn he is looking at, but I'm sure at some point he takes care of himself, if you get my drift. He's like some kind of adolescent who has just figured out how to jerk off. It's really a huge turn-off that he's so immature. He has a ten-year-old son who visits every other weekend. I keep telling him that this isn't good for his son, if he should find this out about his father, but Dave doesn't seem to care enough to stop. I really can't stand it and I've started looking for my own apartment. This must have been what put his ex-wife over the edge as well. He's definitely some kind of an addict."

Kayla was married to her husband, Dean, for five years before she found out that he always had at least one girlfriend on the side and sometimes more. By that time Kayla had two small children and was really scared about getting a divorce. Kayla says, "I always knew that Dean was seductive with all women. We can't go into a restaurant where he doesn't develop a first-name relationship with the waitress, but I didn't pay too much attention to any of that until I found out that he was sleeping with one of my sister's best friends, who unfortunately is also my obstetrician's nurse. So now, of course, my whole family knows. Dean is a really good liar, and he managed to cover up what he was doing. But now that I know, it's so humiliating, and I feel pathetic. When my sister got angry at her friend, the friend said she was far from Dean's first affair. She thought for sure that I knew all about Dean's various relationships. She told my sister that Dean got interested in her when he came with me to the obstetrician before my younger daughter was born. I guess I was in the examining room, and he had a minute to hit on the nurse. She said that he kept calling her and calling her. Finally he convinced her that I wouldn't mind. Dean told her that I understood that he had a high sex drive and that we had an 'open' marriage. Can you believe that?" Kayla is trying to convince Dean to see a therapist because she now believes that he has a sexual addiction. Does he?

I would like to start out by telling you that many psychologists don't believe that there is such a thing as a sex addict. The current thinking is that you cannot become addicted to sex in the same way you can become hooked on drugs or alcohol, and that a behavior such as having sex or eating or gambling does not meet the criteria for a true addiction. Experts do, however, acknowledge compulsive disorders.

Historically, the guy with compulsive sexual behavior has been called many things ranging from a Don Juan and a womanizer to a satyr and a plain old-fashioned pervert. One of the most essential things we can say about the man who is exhibiting compulsive sexual behavior is that he is no longer in control of his behavior; instead it is controlling him. This is the guy who can't stop. He is willing to spend the rent or mortgage money on prostitutes and strip clubs; he is willing to risk alienating loved ones; he may even watch Internet porn at work, willing to take a chance with his job and his reputation.

It seems as though there are a variety of news headlines every day that confirm that these men exist all around us. A recent news story told about an almost fifty-year-old lawyer who was discovered without his clothes on in an empty conference room in a court-house. With him was a fifteen-year-old girl. Almost every day there is some new revelation about one politician after another who has been "outed" for visiting brothels or having affairs or acting out in airport men's rooms. We can understand more about the nature of compulsive behavior whenever we hear stories of successful and ambitious men who are prepared to risk their futures for sexual adventure.

DEFINING SEXUALLY COMPULSIVE BEHAVIOR

If Jean, who ideally would like to have sex a couple of times a week, starts a relationship with Paul, who wants to have sex a couple of times a day, she may wonder, "Is he some kind of sex addict?" But if Jean and Paul break up, and Paul then gets involved with Maria, who regularly wears out her vibrator battery, Maria might think, "If Paul only had a high and low setting, this would be a relationship made in heaven!" In short, one woman's sex addict might be another woman's dream lover.

Before you jump to any conclusions about your guy's sexual behavior, I think you also need to recognize that many people—men and women—are just more adventurous and sexually driven than others. Some relationships also go through stages in which both partners are more interested in sexual experimentation. When Michael and Sophie first met, for example, they simply couldn't get enough of each other. Michael said he liked having sex with

Sophie so much that he wanted to try *everything* with her. They started out by trying every position known to mankind in every place in the apartment. They had sex on the dining room chairs, on the dining room table, and under the dining room table with Michael's hands tied to the table legs. Sophie said she didn't want to do that again because there wasn't really room for her head, and she ended up with a stiff neck. Then Michael brought home sex toys that they could use on each other as well as lacy outfits Sophie could wear that came with ready-made holes in the crotch. Does this behavior make Michael, or Sophie for that matter, sexually compulsive? I don't think so. I think it just describes the kind of high sexuality that often exists in new relationships.

Before you decide your man is a sex addict, also consider this: Men tend to think and fantasize about sex many more times a day than women do. They just seem to be wired that way. In fact, they think about sex more in both positive and negative ways. They have more sexual thoughts that they describe as disturbing or intrusive, as well as more sexual thoughts that impair their concentration. In short, just because he thinks about sex a lot doesn't mean that he is a sex addict.

I also think it's important that women understand that there is a difference between a guy who has a high sex drive and one who acts out compulsively. Example: Some men masturbate a great deal, while some men are compulsive masturbators. This isn't defined by how many times a day they masturbate. It's the idea that instead of masturbating for sexual pleasure, they are masturbating to relieve the anxiety they feel if they don't masturbate. Obsessive and compulsive sexual behavior may indeed relieve anxiety temporarily, but for someone with a true compulsive disorder, the anxiety quickly surfaces again, and the quest for sexual activity continues anew.

There are four main elements that are going to be present in seriously compulsive or addictive sexuality. These are:

1. Out-of-control behavior

Ask yourself: Is he able to control his sexual behavior? For example: If he has a meeting first thing in the morning, can he give up sex or masturbation in order to be on time? Every night at one A.M., instead of snoring peacefully next to you, is he in a tightly closed room in front of a computer screen, watching Internet porn? Is he still there at two A.M.? How about three A.M.? Marnie's husband, who insisted upon having sex with her in a closet while her mother was in a near coma in a nearby hospital bed, also seems to be out of control to me. So does Kayla's husband, Dean—the guy who hit on his pregnant wife's obstetrician's nurse while his wife was in the examining room. I had a male friend who was a self-described alcoholic and sex addict. Until he did so much damage to his body that he could no longer drink and was forced to slow down, he seduced and slept with almost every woman he knew—his wife's therapist, his best friend's fiancée (at her engagement party), just about all of the women in his office, as well as those in the office across the hall. He was the last guy in the world you would think of as a player. He was mild mannered, physically unprepossessing, and not at all sexually creepy. He was also a wonderful guy with a million friends, and I find it very difficult to think of him as somebody who was out of control sexually, but to his several wives, all of whom left him for infidelity, I'm sure that's how he appeared. Ultimately, when he settled down, which he did when he was about fifty, he acknowledged that he considered himself out of control.

2. Continuing the behavior even when there are serious and damaging consequences

The man who spends all his money at strip clubs or runs up his credit cards for phone sex, while his long-suffering wife is in their kitchen cutting coupons and making peanut butter sandwiches for the kids, fits into this category. So does the lawyer who risks disbarment by trying to have sex with a teenager in a courthouse. How about the man who is prepared to lose his wife, children, and sometimes even his job because he can't stop watching Internet porn, even at work? Don't forget about the guy who regularly engages in sex with strangers and is sometimes so caught up in the moment that he forgets about protection from STDs. And who hasn't noticed all those politicians and religious leaders who seem to talk about nothing but "family values" and are then exposed for frequenting various prostitutes and escort services?

I've known several men who put themselves at financial risk with sexually compulsive behavior.

Harry, for example, stayed in bed late every morning having sex with his girlfriend while his business fell apart. He ended up having to deal with actual lawsuits because he ignored what was going on at work.

Ned hired a masseuse through a newspaper ad, figuring that he would get some sex from her. She turned out to be part of a two-person robbery team. Ultimately Ned ended up getting arrested because of something she did, and by the time he got it straightened out it cost him about $50,000 in legal fees.

Steve became so interested in his new secretary that instead of working he would take her out for extended sexual lunches. In the meantime, his office manager was stealing him blind. He ended up having to sell his business to get his financial life back on track.

Anyone who is prepared to take the risk of going broke or making the evening news rather than stop his sexual compulsivity gives new meaning to the phrase "serious and damaging consequences."

3. An overriding preoccupation or obsession with sex

A third test for compulsive behavior has to do with his attitude toward sex. Can he stop thinking about sex? Can he stop figuring out how and when he will next be having it? Is he so involved with Internet porn, for example, that he loses interest in a real life with real activities? Most men will go through periods, particularly in adolescence, when they feel as though they are obsessed with sex. It's also quite normal for men to notice women and think about them sexually much of the time. I teach in a college in Southern California, and many of my male colleagues have confided that when faced with the daily task of teaching young women dressed in halter tops and a variety of other skimpy clothing, they can barely concentrate on their lecture and what they are supposed to be teaching. But there is a difference between thinking about sex and being so obsessed that everything else assumes secondary importance.

4. An increasing need for more and more sexual activity

One of the catchwords used when talking about addictive or compulsive behaviors is *tolerance*. We know, for example, that drug addicts develop a tolerance for what they are using and need to keep increasing the amount in order to get the same high. The same thing is true of the sexually compulsive individual. In other words, the behavior escalates. Tolerance is an important concept because it allows us to differentiate between the guy who is simply going through a phase and the guy whose behavior is out of control.

COMPULSIVE BEHAVIOR THAT DESTROYS RELATIONSHIPS

Sexually compulsive behavior can take different forms, but the three forms that seem to have the most damaging impact on relationships are the following.

He can't stop masturbating.

Compulsive masturbation has always been somewhat linked to pornography. These days, more often than not, that pornography is connected to the Internet. Think about how difficult it must be for a sexual woman to be living with a man who consistently prefers masturbating in front of his computer to making love.

Terri, a young mother, describes her experience. "I don't think anyone would believe me if I told them how much Frank masturbates. Most of the time he masturbates in front of his computer monitor, but he also masturbates in the bed, in the middle of the night when he thinks I'm asleep—which I often am until I feel the bed shaking. I used to always pretend that I was still asleep. Now, I'm so angry that I usually grab the covers and move to the couch. One day last week, I was so annoyed that I kicked him hard before I got out of bed. At one time he used to be embarrassed by what he was doing. Then, he would only masturbate in front of the computer monitor with the door closed when I was in the other room, when he thought I wouldn't notice. By the way, it's hard not to notice when his wastebasket is filled with dirty Kleenex! He still doesn't do it in front of me, but otherwise, he doesn't really seem to care if I'm going to figure it out.

"I have to say that his interest in Internet porn got much worse when I was pregnant. It's true that I was tired and went to bed early. Also, I didn't always want to have sex, particularly in the third trimester, so maybe he felt that justified what he was doing. But now, it's totally out of control. I would complain that we aren't having sex, but what he is doing completely grosses me out, and I don't even want to have anything to do with him anymore. Most of all I worry about when the baby is a little older and starts to notice. I think the porn on the Internet is what really got him started. He would rather spend the night in front of his computer playing with himself than anything I can suggest. I don't know what to do and I think we are definitely heading for a divorce."

Internet porn makes it possible for people to see just about any kind of image that might capture their interest. In fact, research shows that the most common sexual behavior people engage in online is watching porn and masturbating. The most common result of this is that the compulsive Internet porn watcher no longer wants to have sex with his real-life partner. Women who live with men who are compulsive about their sexual Internet activities say that it feels as though the intimacy in their relationships all but disappears. They feel excluded and as though their partners are having affairs. They also sometimes become "grossed out" by the kinds of images that are turning their partners on.

He's made you his favorite sex object.

Ellen divorced her first husband ten years ago because he never stopped wanting sex. She says that she had sex with him as many as three or four times a day, every day, and he always wanted more. Even though it has been years since her divorce, she still has vivid and upsetting memories of his behavior. In fact, she says that she has never gotten over the horror of what it was like to live with him.

"Sometimes I wouldn't be able to figure out why he wanted sex. It certainly wasn't that he needed some kind of sexual release. Many times he would have an orgasm and then minutes later he would start fooling around again. He could get an erection, but it might take him hours before he could have another orgasm—but he would keep trying, and he wanted me to keep trying with him. I guess he was so tired that he needed more stimulation, so he would also ask me to fantasize with him and tell him stories about having sex with other guys or sex with women or sex with the dog—anything that he thought would excite him. Sometimes I would do it just to get the sex over with, but I hated it. If I complained that I couldn't have intercourse because I was sore, he would want me to use my hand or my mouth. I reached the point where I was hiding in the garage or in the basement just to get some peace. He was insatiable. It made no sense to me, but that's the way he was. He also used every event as an opportunity for sex. If I was doing the dishes, he would say that I didn't have to stop what I was doing, he could stand in back of me. Ditto if I was peeling potatoes or making a salad. If I was taking a shower, if I was baking a cake! He loved having sex with me while I was still asleep. Sometimes he would wake me up, but to be honest there would be times when I was so tired I would just sleep through the whole thing. He would want me to combine every activity with sex. It simply became more than I could live with."

Women who have been involved with seemingly insatiable men typically say that they start out feeling flattered and desired, but ultimately feel as though they have become depersonalized objects and that there is no real intimacy or lovemaking. They say that they feel as though they are under attack.

He wants to have sex with just about every woman who walks.

We all know who this guy is: He's the guy who is known all over town for his sexual exploits. He's the neighbor who manages to let you know that he's open for an affair if you are ever in the mood; he's the close friend's husband who tells you that you are his favorite extramarital fantasy; he's the store owner who somehow manages discreetly to let you know that you are a very "special" customer. The thing about the compulsive womanizer is that he is usually a very attractive guy. Sometimes he is very smart; sometimes he is very charming. Often he is a combination of all three, which may be one of the reasons why he is so successful with women. He is fun to know and fun to be with—so long as you are not expecting fidelity and exclusivity.

Fiona, for example, was Daniel's second wife, and when they first got married she really adored him. They were married less than two years and she was pregnant with their first child when she began to suspect that he was having an affair with his assistant, but he always denied everything and managed to convince her that it was her imagination. By the time their second child was born, she could see that her suspicions weren't all in her head. He would come home late every night, and when he was home, he was always "walking the dog." The couple lived in New York City, and when Fiona looked out the window of their apartment, she could see him walk the dog to the corner, where he would grab a taxi and both he and the dog would disappear for hours. She used to worry that he would go someplace and forget to bring the dog home. Weekends, he would make up stories about having to go to his office, and he would vanish. Sometimes these were women Fiona knew, people she had to face regularly. She reached the point where she wouldn't go to any of his work-related events because she was so embarrassed that everybody knew exactly what he was doing. After they got divorced and people began to talk to Fiona, she discovered that he was always sleeping with at least two other women, sometimes three.

Fiona's marriage ended because she eventually started a relationship with a divorced dad in her neighborhood who assumed she was single because she was always alone. When Fiona asked Daniel for a divorce, he went ballistic and accused her of disloyalty. She reminded him of what he had been doing for years, and he said that was different because none of his relationships were serious.

A compulsive womanizer can do a great deal of damage to a woman's sense of self-esteem if she takes him seriously. These guys seem to be designed for short-term relationships. Unfortunately many of them don't know this and seem to invite long-term expectations. On the surface at least, these men often appear to encourage situations in which there are two or more women competing for their attentions. Sometimes these men appear to be sleeping with every woman in town as well as their wives or primary girlfriends. Sometimes these men have a Madonna/whore attitude toward women, and they are having sex with every woman in town except their wives and primary girlfriends. Either way, it's a no-win situation.

INTIMACY ISSUES

It sort of doesn't matter whether the guy in your life is in the next room masturbating in front of Internet porn, pursuing you around the house attempting to have sex with you while you are struggling to complete an important work project, or down on a street corner with his cell phone trying to arrange a sexual tryst with another woman—sexually compulsive men share some common denominators. They almost always have trouble establishing genuinely intimate relationships with women. That's because they have a difficult time seeing women as real people with real needs and real feelings. In short, they tend to depersonalize and sexually objectify women.

I think it's important here that we differentiate true intimate relationships and dependent attachments. While the sexually compulsive guy might have an impossible time treating his significant other as an equal and a real live woman, he is often able to become very dependent on her and expect her to behave like a nurturing mom no matter what he is doing. It's very easy for many women to fall into this emotional trap. Instead of walking away from the guy, they make excuses, and continue to protect and nurture him. This, of course, is part of what codependency is all about.

It has long been accepted that people with addictive and compulsive personalities tend to suffer from feelings of low self-esteem or self-worth. Many believe that the addicted adult is still responding to needs for love and nurturing that were not met in childhood. If you were to talk to many of the women who are in relationships with addicted men, no matter what that addiction might be, you would often hear them describe the men in their lives as needy and dependent.

SUGGESTIONS FOR WOMEN IN RELATIONSHIPS WITH SEXUALLY COMPULSIVE MEN

1. Accept the fact that you did not create and are not causing his attitude.

It's not your fault that your significant other is hooked on pornography and masturbation; it's not your fault if your significant other is compulsively unfaithful; it's not even your fault that you can't lean down to put a roast in the oven without your partner trying to nail you. Whatever he is doing is coming from a place in his own psyche that has little or nothing to do with what is taking place between the two of you.

2. Realize that his behavior has little or nothing to do with who you are or how you are.

He's not watching Internet porn because you are undesirable, and he is not being compulsively unfaithful because there is something wrong with you as a partner. I don't know how to tell you this, but even if you are his favored sexual object, this also has much more to do with him and his sexual journey than it does with you or what you are wearing.

3. Stop thinking that external circumstances are going to alter his behavior.

Women involved with sexually compulsive men keep thinking that a miracle will happen and he will change. They think that if the other woman or women in his life were to leave, for example, he would change; they think that if all the porn shops would go out of business, he would change; they think that once they have a family, he will change. It doesn't happen. Unless there are drastic changes in his approach to sex, his behavior is not going to change. If you hide his pornographic DVDs or magazines, he will get others. If you disconnect his Internet connection, he will find another hook-up. Any changes in his attitude are going to have to come from him.

4. Stop playing detective.

If you are inclined to go through his wallet, pockets, computer, and bookcases looking for proof of his sexual behavior, don't do it.

Once you know what's going on, you know. You don't need more proof, you don't need to reinforce your discomfort, and you don't need to turn into a crazy person.

5. Be honest about your sexual feelings, needs, and reactions.

Don't do things you don't want to do sexually. Set your boundaries and stick with them. Don't agree to activities that turn you off; don't pretend to enjoy sexual conversations about fantasies that gross you out. Also don't fake orgasms just to please him. In short, don't go along with his tendency to depersonalize his sexual partners. You are a real, honest woman, so start behaving accordingly.

6. Do find somebody with whom you can talk.

Hiding his behavior isn't going to help you. Find somebody you trust in whom you can confide. If this person is a professional counselor or therapist, all the better. Many women who are involved with sexually compulsive men have a tendency to go into denial or hide what's going on. They feel ashamed and embarrassed about discussing intimate sexual details. This attitude isn't going to help you in the long run. These are the times when it really helps to have a trained professional.

7. Do insist on safer sex practices.

In this day and age, it seems redundant to say the obvious, but: If you believe he is having sex with multiple partners, don't have sex with him without taking precautions against STDs.

SOME COMMON QUESTIONS ABOUT SEXUALLY COMPULSIVE MEN

Can he change his behavior?

Of course he can, but he has to want to change. This is something he has to do for himself; you can't do it for him. Many sexually compulsive men recognize that their behavior is destructive to others as well as themselves. They realize that they have engaged in inappropriate as well as risky sexual behavior. Some actually feel quite tormented by what they are doing. Compulsive masturbators, for example, often feel guilty and ashamed, as does the man who lies to his significant others about where he has been and who he has been with.

Is there any medication a guy can take for compulsive sexual behavior?

Some doctors recommend drugs like Prozac, which can alter a guy's sexual responses. I would only suggest medication for a guy who really wants to change and who has tried every other method of altering his behavior because some of these medications may lead to other forms of sexual dysfunction. A man who chooses this route needs to be working with a doctor who is very sensitive to the sexual side effects and who has a sophisticated understanding of how to appropriately tweak medication dosage.

Can you spot a sexually compulsive guy when you first meet him?

It's not always possible on the first meeting, but many times the sexually compulsive man does give you some hints about his interests.

Here are some clues:

Does he sexualize every situation? If you are talking about a completely nonsexual subject, for example, does he find a way to put in a sexual innuendo?

Does he test your sexual tolerance levels? Does he introduce sexual subjects in a way in which he appears to be checking out how accepting and understanding you are about high levels of sexual interest?

Does he talk excessively about his sexual adventures and interests? Does he have too many stories about ex-lovers and sex?

Does he put down other men for what they do sexually? This may seem strange, but sexually compulsive men sometimes seem to enjoy having conversations of the "pot calling the kettle scorched" variety.

Is it ever possible to have a sexual relationship with a sexually compulsive guy?

Of course it is. In fact, you might be able to have a very good and exciting sexual relationship. The difficulties occur when you try to have a genuinely intimate, committed, long-term relationship with one of these guys. In the short term, as long as you are self-protective and have realistic expectations, the sex can be great. They've often had a great deal of sex and are experienced, competent lovers.

How can you tell if a guy is hooked on Internet porn?

It would appear that more and more men (and women) are spending larger and larger portions of their lives watching pornography on the Internet. The thing about many men who are involved with the Internet is that what they are doing is not immediately obvious. The activities they are involved with are primarily solitary and unless you access their computers, you are clueless about what they are viewing or how they are viewing it. Many men feel guilty about what they are viewing and don't talk about it; others realize that some women might find their viewing habits creepy, so they don't talk about it. Unless you ask or somehow bring up the subject of time spent on the Internet, for whatever reason, you can't get a true sense of what's going on. Having said that, however, usually if you start dating a guy or spending any time where he lives, you can get a sense of what he is doing by how he handles his computer and how he makes sure you don't see what he has on the screen. Women I've spoken to who have been in relationships with compulsive Internet porn watchers say that there are several clues.

- He is more interested in getting back to his computer than he is in being with you.
- He limits sleepovers at your place and always seems anxious to return to his own space.
- When you stay over at his home, you discover that he is up early in the morning or late at night at the computer, and you don't think it's work-related or that he is a news junkie.
- He gets nervous if you go near his computer or changes the screen when you come into the room.

A SPECIAL WARNING ABOUT A RELATIONSHIP MODEL TO BE AVOIDED

Some of the women who are attracted to sexually compulsive men are women who might themselves be "addicted" to love. They then form relationships that can best be described in the following way:

"When the Sex Junkie Meets the Love Junkie." This is a terrible relationship model. In these relationships, the guy is usually interested in pursuing a variety of sexual objects and interests while the woman is interested in only one thing: getting approval and love from the man who is incapable of giving her what she needs. If you have a tendency to fall into this kind of relationship, it's really important that you realize what you are doing and get some appropriate professional guidance. Many women have wasted years of their lives standing by guys who act out sexually. Do whatever you need to do to develop a more independent attitude!

WHAT RESOURCES AND HELP ARE AVAILABLE

If you are involved with a man who feels that he is sexually compulsive and wants to change, there are several things he can do, starting with individual therapy and/or counseling. In addition, if you are both committed to working on the relationship, it might be a good idea to see a couples' counselor together. There are also several twelve step recovery programs patterned after Alcoholics Anonymous. These include Sex Addicts Anonymous, Sexaholics Anonymous, Sex and Love Addicts Anonymous, and Sexual Recovery Anonymous. Information about these organizations and others can be found online and provide support as well as information about literature and meetings.

There are also several twelve step programs for the friends and family of sexual compulsives. These include Codependents of Sexual Addiction (COSA) and S-Anon.

8

Kinky and Compulsive

Before I became a sex therapist, I worked for the United States Postal Service for several years. For much of this time I carried mail. When you are a mail carrier, and you are a woman, you are the target for, as my friends used to say, "every wienie wagger in town." I remember that I couldn't believe the risks that men would take to expose themselves to me as well as the other female carriers.

Once I was walking down a street doing my route, and a man pulled his car up to the curb, opened the window, and waved a map at me. He yelled, "Mail lady! Mail lady! Could you come over here? I need some directions." When I got next to his car, he pulled the map away from his lap. His fly was unzipped and his erect penis was sticking out. Some of my fellow mail carriers told me at the time that I gained a place in the postal hall of fame by saying, "You need directions? Why don't you put your hand around it and move it up and down?!"

After I left the post office, I sort of forgot all my experiences with men whose kinks involved exposing themselves until one day several years ago when I was driving to a convention at a hotel in Long Beach, California. A guy in a sports car pulled up next to me on the freeway and started pacing me. (How annoying, not to mention dangerous.) When I looked over at him, he had somehow managed to put a leg up on the seat. He had his fly open and he was stroking his erect penis so that I could see it through the open window of his car. He followed me all the way to an outside parking lot in Long Beach. I sat there for a second trying to decide what to do. In the meantime, he wasted no time in getting out of his car and walking through the lot toward me. His fly was open and his penis was hanging out. No one else in the parking lot even noticed him!

He walked up to my car, opened the passenger door, and said, "I have to jack off right now." At this point my mouth was hanging open, I was so shocked, and by now, I'm sure you've also figured out that very little shocks me. All I could think of to say was, "Just don't get it on the sheepskin seat covers. They're new." "Don't worry," he replied, "I brought my own paper towel." And he proceeded to ejaculate with one stroke. Then comes the really unbelievable part—he reached into his other pocket and pulled out a twenty-dollar bill and threw it at me and said, "Thanks." I swear this is a true story. I asked him, "How often do you do this?" And he said, "Eight to ten times a day, but I only pay some of them."

Both of these guys—the one who asked for directions and the one in the parking lot—provide concrete examples of what it means for a man to be kinky as well as so driven by his sexual compulsions that he is prepared to take seemingly insane risks. The technical term for a sexual kink, by the way, is *paraphilia*. The closest thing we have to a definition of *paraphilia* is "strange love" or "abnormal love." The list of possible paraphilias is extensive, beginning with abasiophilia, which is an attraction to orthopedic devices such as braces or crutches, and continues on through zoophilia, which is a sexual attraction to animals. It is far more common for a man to have paraphilic interests than it is for a woman. (I've seen estimates that place it at twenty to one, male to female.) Some paraphilias are more common than others, and many, of course, are illegal. Now that we've learned the formal word, I'm going to stop using it all the time and rely on the more familiar "kinky." The following are the most common kinky behaviors.

Sadism is the need to hurt or humiliate another person. Masochism is the need to be hurt or humiliated.

Sadism and masochism tend to go together. In consensual sexual sadism, a man or woman who has sadistic tendencies will pair up with a partner with masochistic interests and agree to do an S&M scene—a role-playing activity such as doctor and patient, pirate and wench, or dominatrix and slave, in which each person has a stereotyped role. These roles are agreed on beforehand and include a "safe word"—a phrase that one of the participants can say if they want to get out of the role immediately. Consensual sexual sadists rarely suggest any activities that will draw blood or result in permanent injury or disfigurement, but of course there are exceptions, and sometimes people do get hurt. I have known women who have been introduced to S&M by experienced practitioners and they were okay with it. Many women, however, hear that a man is into S&M and they run screaming in the other direction. One man with kinky interests, for example, shocked his wife of ten years by taking her to an S&M dungeon. When she realized what was going on, she became very upset. He in turn became angry. "If you would just stop crying long enough to give it a chance," he said, "you might like it." Nobody was surprised when the marriage ended shortly thereafter.

Every now and then, a woman tells me that she was unfortunate enough to meet a nonconsensual sexual sadist. In these encounters, typically a woman goes to bed with a man she doesn't know that well, presuming that they are going to make love. Then, during the course of the sexual encounter, he pulls her hair, smacks her on the butt, bites her, or does other aggressive behaviors that she doesn't like and to which she hasn't given her consent. This can be very frightening and upsetting. If this happens to you, it goes without saying that you need to voice your disapproval loudly and immediately.

Sexual masochists derive sexual gratification from being hurt or humiliated by their partners. The spread of sexual masochism has seemingly increased exponentially in the past few years and it appears to have become far more complex. Many sexual masochists, by the way, are male. These are the kind of guys who cheerfully pay to put on dog collars while dominatrix types lead them around on leashes and tell them that they are worthless.

In the world of consensual S&M, there are a variety of other terms used to describe these practices, such as B&D (bondage and discipline) and D&S (domination and submission). They are frequently grouped together using the initials BDSM. Other terms used include "top," referring to the more dominant partner, and "bottom," when describing the more submissive. Some participants in BDSM always play the same role, while others switch regularly.

Fetishism is the sexual attraction to inanimate objects such as shoes or fabrics.
Partialism is a sexual attraction to a part of the body we don't normally think of as an erogenous zone, such as the feet or earlobes.

When I teach my Human Sexuality class at Cal State Fullerton, I usually talk about fetishism and partialism at the same time.

There is shoe fetishism and foot partialism, for example, and they often go together. People tend to say "foot fetish" because it sounds alliterative, but technically it's not correct.

There are varying degrees of shoe fetishes. These can range from the small—he wants you to wear high heels every time you have sex—to the more extreme—his preferred spot to ejaculate is in your most expensive pair of sandals. Some men want to buy a variety of women's shoes and keep them in a special closet. Every weekend they decide, "Who should I date tonight?" and then take out a pair of shoes and after some extended fantasy time, masturbate and ejaculate on the shoes.

Other men can only get sexually excited if they see the woman who has worn the shoes. That means they sometimes resort to stealing shoes in settings in which women are likely to take them off, such as airplanes or movie theaters. In these cases, the shoes do not necessarily have to be sexy-looking. True shoe fetishists tend to be attracted by a certain type of shoe—the traditional black, stiletto-heeled "do me" shoe with a low throat that exposes toe cleavage. Foot partialists, on the other hand, may steal stinky gym shoes, or other shoes that we would not think of as sexy. Some of them are into it primarily for the odor.

Sometimes a foot partialist will want to have sex in a way that actually involves the foot. Maybe he wants to stick his big toe into a woman's vagina. Maybe he wants a woman to rub her foot on his penis. Maybe he wants to put his penis between a woman's big toe and second toe and masturbate.

I use the example of shoe fetishists and foot partialists because these are very common, but there are other types of fetishes. One of the earlier explanation of fetishes that I read was that people become attracted to inanimate objects or fabrics that feel good, like leather or silk or feathers. I have not always found this to be the case. Some people have a fetish for rubber, of all things. I remember talking to a female acquaintance several years ago, and she said, "I have a new boyfriend. We went to Las Vegas. Want to see the pictures?" And I said, "Sure." I was looking at the pictures, and she and her boyfriend were wearing evening clothes, and I said, "Those outfits look kind of weird. Why?" And she said, "Because they're made of rubber. That's a rubber evening gown I'm wearing and he's wearing a rubber tuxedo. We went to Las Vegas to attend a conference of people who have a fetish for rubber clothing."

Transvestic fetishism, also known as cross-dressing, is when someone wears clothing usually associated with the opposite sex for the specific purpose of becoming sexually aroused.

Believe it or not, there are many reasons why a man might dress in women's clothing other than because he is a transvestite. Some male bonding groups such as fraternities require men to dress in women's clothes as part of their initiation because it is humiliating. I know this is also true of some fraternal groups such as the Shriners and the Bohemian Club. But true male cross-dressers or transvestites dress in women's clothes because for them it is a huge turn-on.

Contrary to popular belief, most transvestites are not gay and many are married heterosexual men. I should mention here that I have known several women who were happily involved with cross-dressers, claiming that they were great guys and good husbands and fathers. Also, some women find it really sexy to see a man dressed in lingerie.

Exhibitionism is the need to expose your genitals to an unsuspecting person.
Voyeurism is the need to watch people getting undressed or having sex. It's the flip side of exhibitionism.

Nonconsensual exhibitionism and voyeurism can be highly problematic behaviors. First of all, they are illegal, although in the case of a voyeur, it's often difficult to prove what he was looking at or seeing if he is found sneaking through someone's yard. Usually when they get arrested, it's for trespassing or loitering. Exhibitionists, as most of us have experienced, can flash their way through the world, often eluding law enforcement for years before their behavior escalates to the point where they get caught. Typically by the time you've been able to contact authorities and the police arrive, the exhibitionist is long gone.

Most exhibitionists and voyeurs tend to be young—teens and early twenties, so you can forget about the stereotype of the dirty old man flasher. They also tend (no surprise here) to have low social skills and poor peer relationships. The big question is: Are they dangerous? Will the typical exhibitionist or voyeur escalate to the point that he gets violent or assaults a victim? This is a good question, and authorities believe that only about 10 percent of exhibitionists and voyeurs will progress to the point where they assault a victim. Let's face it—sooner or later, some voyeurs and/or exhibitionists are no longer going to be content by just looking through an open window while masturbating. Some of these men are going to test that window to see if it's unlocked and ultimately end up standing over a woman while masturbating. The problem is that we don't know which of these men will escalate. All I can say is that if a man has several paraphilias, rather than one (in other words, if he is both an exhibitionist and a voyeur), and if his behavior is escalating, there is a real chance that he will pose a potential danger to a victim.

Bestiality and zoophilia both have to do with sex with animals.

Bestiality describes someone who has sex with animals, although he might actually prefer a human partner. Put another way, some men who grew up in rural areas had their first sexual experience with an animal because there were no potential human partners. Zoophiles (known as "zoos"), on the other hand, think of an animal as their lover or sexual partner. In other words, zoophilia is a sexual orientation to animals rather than people.

Sex with animals is much more common than many of us think. It takes many forms. There are some countries in which you could watch a live sex show featuring women having sex with animals. Sex with animals can take the form of watching a sex show, having an animal lick you after sex, masturbating with or on an animal, buying an animal that has been trained to have sex with a person, or actually falling in love with an animal and believing that animal is your sexual partner or soul mate.

I once knew a guy who told me that his ex-girlfriend had a dog, and after the two of them had intercourse, the dog would lick the guy's penis. I don't know what to think about this. I also once knew a woman who lived in a high-rise with her boyfriend and a small dog. We were having lunch one day with a group of people, and someone asked her, "You know, you and your boyfriend are gone all day at work, and you live in this apartment. Doesn't your dog get lonely all day?" And she said, "Yeah, that's a problem, so whichever one of us gets home from work first masturbates the dog to make him feel better." And she was serious! I think every person sitting at that table just about choked on lunch at that point.

Sex with animals is actually a culturally universal behavior. It has existed in every culture and historical period. It is also, as one might imagine, illegal. One of the main objections that animal rights organizations raise about having sex with animals is that, like children, animals cannot consent to sexual activity. The rational that "zoos" use to counter this objection is often along the lines of "Of course my dog is agreeing to have sex with me. . . . If he didn't agree to it, he would bite me!"

Frotteurism is about inappropriate touching.

I'm told that any woman who has regularly ridden the New York City subway system is intimately aware of this behavior, even if she didn't know what to call it. *Frotteurism* is the technical word used to describe the man who gets his thrills by rubbing his body (specifically his genitals) against the body of an unsuspecting and nonconsenting person. The term *frotteurism* is also used to describe someone who fondles the genitals of another person in a public place.

Pedophilia is a sexual interest and attraction to children.

Pedophiles pose a real danger to society. Fortunately, most of them restrict their interest in children to fantasy and viewing pornography. Nonetheless, suffice it to say, if you look on your boyfriend's or husband's computer and see images of real children in sexual poses, it is illegal to even possess them.

Other kinky behaviors

There are a wide variety of other kinky behaviors including necrophilia that I'm not even going to go into. I think the Internet, which contains millions of images of unusual sexual behavior, has made it possible for many people to engage in their normal curiosity—for example, to perhaps see someone getting an enema.

It's possible to go on the Internet and, with a few key strokes, see scenes of people defecating on each other, having large objects stuck into the anus, dressing up as infants, piercing their genitals, and suspending themselves from rings pierced into their breasts and genitals. As recently as twenty years ago, you couldn't even buy pictures of this stuff in the dirtiest adult bookstore in town. (I know because I tried.) But now, men, women, *and* children can go on the Internet and have a choice of photos. With all of these people fixated on their computer monitors, it stands to reason that some men viewing this on the Internet are going to want to include some of these behaviors in their bedroom activity, either in fact or in fantasy. Also, there are a fair number of men who are into anal eroticism—inserting larger and larger objects into their rectums for the purpose of sexual pleasure. You will have to figure out whether your partner's interest in this is just a gross-out curiosity or a long-standing sexual compulsion.

WHEN DOES KINKINESS BECOME A PROBLEM?

Kinky behavior differs from so-called normal sexual behavior in terms of quantity, not quality. This means that paraphilias are extensions of normal behaviors and curiosities. Here's an example. Let's say you had a nice dinner at home and decided to walk your dog. There you are, standing on a public sidewalk, and you look at a house and there's a big picture window that offers a good view of someone's living room, and there's a naked woman standing there in the picture window! Admit it, you'd look! We'd all look! That doesn't mean you're a voyeur. When confronted with a naked person, most of us would stare.

I remember one time when I was teaching high school (a sordid part of my past I'd prefer to forget). The classroom I was using had windows that looked down on a parking lot. Suddenly one of the students looked out the window and yelled, "There are two dogs down there having sex in the back of a pickup truck!" All of the students ran over to the window (I did, too). This is normal curiosity. It doesn't mean those students wanted to have sex with animals. Paraphilias, then, are extreme extensions of normal desires, impulses, or curiosity.

There are several criteria that psychologists use to determine whether paraphilic interests have become so extreme that they may reach the level of a full-blown mental disorder. Some of those criteria are:

1. Does the behavior involve a human partner?

Some psychologists believe that any behavior that does not involve a human partner is highly problematic. I don't always agree with that. For example, there are many people who have an auto-erotic sexual orientation—they only want to masturbate and have sex with themselves. While I wouldn't advise any woman to get romantically involved with a guy like this, I don't know if this kind of behavior always belongs in the category of a full-blown mental disorder—so long as the man isn't trying to manipulate, fool, or hurt others.

2. Is the behavior statistically normal—that is, do most people do it?

While psychologists typically use this criterion to distinguish whether sexual behavior is acceptable, in fact, we don't have a really good idea today about what percent of the population participates in kinky activities. I have looked for statistics about this all over the place, and the only thing I can feel confident about stating is this: They are more common than they used to be, and they are more common that you think. I think we have room for a great deal of diversity in sexual response, and it's difficult to definitively decide what's normal and what's not. It wasn't that long ago, for example, that some of the most common sexual behaviors (including oral sex) were considered pathological.

3. Is the behavior illegal?

Just because it's illegal under some circumstances doesn't make it abnormal. It just makes it dangerous. Let's face it, if you're a guy who wants to run around naked in his own home or in a nudist colony, for that matter, chances are no one is going to care. Whereas if you run around all over town exposing your genitals to children and little old ladies, you've got a huge legal problem as well as a possible psychological one.

Some experts divide paraphilias into two classifications— coercive versus noncoercive, or consensual versus nonconsensual. Behaviors such as mutual sadism and masochism (an S&M "scene") are entered into voluntarily by the participants. On the other hand, behaviors like nonconsensual voyeurism and exhibitionism have a "victim" and are therefore illegal. Illegal/coercive/nonconsensual paraphilias put the perpetrator at risk of arrest and, by extension, they put you at risk if your partner practices them.

4. Does the behavior have an addictive or compulsive component?

Does it take more and more frequent instances of the behavior to get the same amount of sexual thrill? Does the man seem to engage in the behavior as much to reduce anxiety as to get sexual enjoyment? Does he have to do more extreme versions of the sexual behavior to achieve the same level of sexual satisfaction? These are interesting questions. Many men with kinky interests definitely have a tendency to step up their activities over time. The guy who starts out small by unzipping his fly in the privacy of his own car on a darkened street can quickly escalate into being the kind of guy who gets a thrill out of exposing himself to female mail carriers on a regular basis.

5. Does the behavior cause personal distress?

There are many men who are upset and conflicted by what they perceive to be their kinky sexual behavior. This is particularly true of those guys whose regular day-to-day worlds appear to be at direct odds with their secret sexual activities. We've all seen headlines discussing the activities of men who spend their days as evangelical preachers or conservative politicians deriding sexual behavior that they themselves are engaging in regularly. How conflicted they must be!

On a much less complex level, think about the many men who like to dress in women's clothing because it gives them a sexual thrill. A fair number of these men are "out" to their families; they are comfortable cross-dressing in their own homes and feel okay about it. Some regularly go out in public dressed in drag and are okay with doing this. But there are also many transvestites who are still "in the closet." Whether they are married or single, they may keep a few pieces of women's lingerie hidden in a secret place. Maybe they fondle them or masturbate with them once in a while, or maybe they wear women's panties under their clothes to work or when they go out with family or friends. Either way, they would be absolutely mortified if anyone found out about this. Often they live in fear that their secret will be exposed to the world. A guy like this may try to stop the behavior, but he may find he is unable to give it up. These men are not okay with what they perceive to be their "deviant" and "uncontrollable" desires. Sometimes these men seek psychological help. The guy who is intensely conflicted or distressed by his kinkiness may be unable to be honest with his romantic partner. This can create even more relationship problems.

6. Does the behavior interfere with other life goals?

All of us have both short-term and long-term goals. Short-term goals include "Just let me get to the weekend." Some long-term goals include: graduate from college, get a good job in a field I enjoy, buy a house, have children.

People whose involvement with kinky behavior is in direct conflict with their long-term goals include the student who skips final exams in order to stay home and have sex with the dog. Another example is the husband who regularly disappoints his wife and brings her to the brink of divorce. In one instance, for example, she was waiting for him in a restaurant with family members to celebrate an anniversary. He never showed up because he said he was compelled to stay home and rig up a device to deliver electrical shocks to his nipples and penis while he masturbated for several hours in a row. It happens, and I've heard all of the above.

CLUBS AND ORGANIZATIONS FOR THOSE WHO LIKE KINKINESS

In most large cities there are a wide variety of fetish clubs, or dungeons, designed to fulfill the needs of those who prefer kinky sex. If you were to visit one of these clubs, you might see exhibitionist couples engaging in sexual activities while voyeuristic individuals gather around and masturbate. Walk around, and you might spot spanking benches and ventilated coffins, as well as people pretending to be dogs or horses. You might discover that these clubs have vendors who are selling a variety of sexual toys and paraphernalia ranging from dildos and chastity cages for male genitals to stiletto heels and whips; you might learn that they are sponsoring a series of lectures on subjects like "nontraditional bondage" and how to flog a partner in ways that can create fear and excitement without causing damage. Many of the people who regularly visit these dungeons appear to be spectacularly ordinary and middle class.

One of the main things about these clubs is the emphasis on "consensual" activities. Voyeurs focus on exhibitionists; dominants search out submissives; and most of them seem to prefer to play by specified rules, which include not causing any physical harm.

WHAT CAUSES AN INTEREST IN KINKY BEHAVIOR?

There have been many theories put forth about what causes people to have these comparatively unusual sexual interests. In general, we only know a couple of things for sure. One is that paraphilic interests start very early—well before puberty. Men who cross-dress start stealing their mother's or sister's clothes around the age of eight. Masochism is perhaps the paraphilia about which we know the most. Therefore, most of the psychological theories about causes of paraphilic interests have to do with causes of masochistic interests. Here are some of the theories:

I. Psychoanalytic/Freudian theory

This is the idea that men with paraphilic interests were probably sexually abused themselves as children. We do find that if you survey a group of people with kinky interests and compare them with a sample of people who don't have these interests, you will find a much higher incidence of child-adult sexual experiences.

2. Learning theory

When I was in grammar school, corporal punishment was not only common, it was often considered desirable! The theory here is that if an eight-year-old boy is put over a woman's knee and spanked, he would associate the physical pain of the spanking with the arousal of feeling of his penis rubbing against a woman's lap.

3. Social roles theory

This is the idea that if a man has a very high-powered position in business in which he is always in control, he may need to relax by letting someone else have complete control of him—namely an S&M mistress or dominatrix. Several years ago, a friend introduced me to a dominatrix who at the time had a dungeon in Southern California. I interviewed her for my radio show. She said that most of her clients were lawyers or businessmen—guys who were obviously huge control freaks in their work lives.

4. Biological theory

When you are in a highly aroused state, your brain secretes chemicals called *endorphins*, which are pleasure-causing, painkilling chemicals. The idea here is that people who are into S&M are wired a little differently, and they convert pain signals into pleasure more readily than the rest of us do.

5. Cross-cultural theory

There are people who are known as "modern primitives," who travel to other countries and observe religious rites, many of which involve bondage or body mortification. They then bring these practices back to the United States and use them for sexual purposes. Interestingly enough, in the culture in which they are practiced, these rites are typically used for anti-sexual purposes and were initially intended to mortify the body so the practitioner either wouldn't feel sexual impulses or would be better able to atone for perceived sexual transgressions.

An example of a practice that modern primitives have incorporated into their sexuality can be seen in the holy men of India known as Sadhus. These holy men practiced stretching of their penile tissues so they wouldn't be distracted by sexual feelings. Modern primitives might do the same thing because it turns them on sexually. Some say that all the complex body piercing, which we now see everywhere, evolved from this movement.

My first introduction to this concept was several years ago when I was shooting a show for Playboy television and a guy in California rented us his house for the shoot. This guy was one of these modern primitives. We weren't supposed to be looking around the house at all of his personal stuff, but you couldn't help it. He had some really bizarre artwork on his walls. I remember a picture of a woman with weights hanging off her clitoris and a picture of a man with a rope tied around his penis and pulling it into his rectum. One picture showed a person with small balloons pinned into the skin of his back. People were throwing darts at the balloons and trying to break them, like a carnival game. It was a human dartboard!

6. Controlled pain theory

A friend of mine who was really into S&M explained this theory to me, and it actually makes sense to me. He said that being human always involves some kind of pain, whether it's psychological or physical. It could be caused by childhood trauma or loss at any age. People deal with their pain in very different ways. Some use alcohol or drugs; others sublimate pain through artistic expression. There are people, however, who deal with their pain by either hurting themselves physically or having others do it. The thinking goes something like this: "The only solution for uncontrollable pain is controllable pain."

DISCOVERING THAT HE IS KINKIER THAN HE APPEARS

I once interviewed a professional dominatrix and I asked her about the most unusual client she had ever known. She said, "That has to be the guy I called 'Peacock Man.'" I should add here that this is by no means the grossest or weirdest sexual story I have ever heard; it just happens to be the one I have unsuccessfully been trying to scrape out of my brain cells for ten years. "Peacock Man" would come in her house dressed like a normal businessman, take off his clothes, and crawl around the floor on his hands and knees. He would want her to ride on his back and whip him, which is not so unusual, but while this was going on, he wanted to have a dozen long peacock feathers stuck into his rectum so that they stuck up like a peacock's tail.

At this point, I should also tell you about the most perverted man I ever knew. His name was Bob. He and his wife were friends of friends of mine. When we met, he and I kind of hit it off, and we would have lunch together every now and then. Once he started to trust me, he told me a little bit about his "extracurricular" activities. You've heard of heterosexual, homosexual, and bisexual? I think Bob was omnisexual. Literally everything would turn him on. If he saw a documentary that said, "And then the amoeba divides," his eyes would get all big and he'd say, "Where? Can I watch?"

Bob was into sticking sharp objects into his genitals and suspending himself by pulleys from rings in his scrotum. Obviously I didn't participate in these activities with him, but he showed me Polaroids. One of the photos showed his scrotum stretched onto a wooden cutting board, with objects like corn-on-the-cob holders stuck in it. He told me that his wife of twenty-plus years didn't want to have sex with him anymore, and I said, "If it involved D-rings and fondue forks, I wouldn't either!" Nevertheless, he and his wife stayed married, and when I spoke to her years later, I realized that she was deeply in love with him. So yes, it is possible to love someone kinky even if you no longer want to have sex with him.

The point of all this is that there are a wide variety of kinky men walking around among us. They date; they get married; they become fathers. Some of these men are very open about their sexual preferences. Others keep these interests deeply hidden, exposing them only to a chosen few. You might even be dating someone with paraphilic interests and not find out about it until after you are already involved.

Take the example of Beth, a forty-two-year-old copywriter, who met Benjamin, a forty-six-year-old divorced lawyer, on one of the better-known Internet dating services. She thought he was just great! He liked everything she liked—film, concerts, good restaurants. They shared an interest in politics and supported the same environmental causes. He understood that Beth's two teenage sons were her first priority because he had a twenty-two-year-old daughter he adored. After about a month of dating, they had sex. Beth said he was a very gentle, loving, affectionate, and attentive lover. After a couple of months of dating, they went away together for a long weekend in the country. It was idyllic and featured long walks, leisurely bubble baths, and romantic sex. The night after they returned, Benjamin asked Beth to come to his apartment for dinner. He said he had something to tell her and something he wanted to show her.

When Beth arrived at Benjamin's apartment, he got her a glass of wine and sat her down. "I really like you," he said, "and I think we could have a very good relationship. But I want to be honest and there is something you have to know before we go any further. Please come with me."

Beth didn't know what to expect as Benjamin led her into his bedroom and said, "I want you to see my closet." For a second, Beth felt panic. What was he going to show her? But when he opened the door, all she saw were rows of neatly hung women's clothes and shelves filled with shoes, hats, scarves, and wigs. *Wigs?*

Beth's mouth was as open as the closet door. "I like to wear women's clothes," Ben said. "I hope this is something that you can handle."

Beth said that there had been nothing in his behavior that might have made her suspect his interest in cross-dressing. As much as Beth liked him, she ultimately decided that she didn't want to have a long-term relationship with him. She said that she could have probably managed to go along with his cross-dressing, but she would be terrified if friends or members of her family found out—what they would say or think?

Occasionally, a woman will find out about a man's more kinky sexual interests on the first date. Other times, it may be years before she figures them out or even realizes that they exist. Some men are more honest and want to share them with the women they love; others prefer to keep these interests secret and hidden. Many men want to tell their wives or girlfriends about their sexual interests, but, as weird as it may seem, some never get up the courage and may go through a lifetime without bringing it up on their own. Men who are involved with organizations devoted to paraphilic interests such as S&M clubs frequently spend time discussing this issue of how to tell their significant others. Everyone agrees there is no easy way. In a perfect world, two people with perfectly meshing kinks would find each other, but that's a rarity if not a downright impossibility.

Nonetheless, if you talk to people who visit clubs or events designed for fetishists, you would discover that there are a fair number of couples who get involved in these activities together and appear to have worked out satisfying ways of incorporating this into their relationship.

DECISIONS YOU HAVE TO MAKE FOR YOURSELF

If you meet a man you're attracted to, and you discover that he has some kinky interests, you might be confused about what to do next. Let's say you go to a friend's barbecue and one of the guests brings a newcomer, a really nice guy named Theo. Like you, Theo is interested in local politics, so you have things to talk about. He asks you out; you say yes. After a couple of dates, Theo lets it drop, almost casually, that he sometimes visits a fetish club. He tells you that he never has sex with anybody there, so he has no fear of any kinds of STDs, but he does watch other people having sex, and he considers it a huge turn-on. He says he was introduced to the club by another friend with masochistic tendencies. Theo says that his friend is also worried about the possibility of STDs so, like Theo, he also never has sex. His friend, however, does wear a dog collar and likes to get on all fours and be led around by a dominatrix, who sometimes uses a whip on him. Theo assures you that it's all a big game and that his friend is never actually hurt.

As you listen to Theo talking, you have several concerns.

You wonder whether you are hearing the whole story. Is it true that Theo never has sex when he visits these clubs? You also wonder whether Theo is telling you the whole truth about "his friend." Is it possible that there is no friend? Is it possible that the person who is being led around by a dominatrix is Theo himself, and he's talking to you about this so that he can find out how you will react?

These are real concerns. If Theo has unprotected sex with strangers in fetish dungeons, you need to think long and hard about what that means in terms of the possibilities of sexually transmitted diseases. Also, if Theo is using the ruse of a masochistic friend in order to get your reactions to sexual behavior, you do need to wonder whether there will be further secrets.

You like Theo, but you are basically turned off by what he told you. If you have absolutely no interest in anything Theo said to you about his turn-ons, and you never expect to have any interest, then this is probably not a sexual relationship that was meant to be. You both deserve partners who are on the same sexual page.

You wonder whether Theo's kinky interests will escalate over time. This is always a real possibility. A great deal depends on Theo's age. Quite often, men who are mildly interested in experimental sexuality when they are younger do find that they need more and more stimulation as their testosterone declines. Another issue to take into account is how often Theo is acting on his kinkier interests and whether it has already escalated. Somebody who visits an S&M dungeon once every month or two presents a completely different picture from somebody who is hanging out there two or three times a week or more.

You wonder: Can he be cured or treated so that his kinkiness will go away? I think the answer here is no. For the most part, paraphilic interests begin so early in life that they basically become part of an individual's personality. I recently attended a lecture given by Jack Morin, a Ph.D. who has done a fair amount of research into this question. I have known Jack for a long time and I really respect his knowledge and experience. In terms of paraphilias, he has what he calls the "roach motel" theory. Remember that old commercial from years ago—"Roaches check in, but they don't check out"? Similarly kinky turn-ons check in, but they don't check out. Based on our current knowledge, you are not going to rid someone of their kinky interests. In fact, when someone tries to repress these interests, they often become more powerful. There have been many attempts to "cure" people of paraphilias. Methods used include social skills training, aversion therapy (not good with guys who are into S&M), empathy training, sex therapy and use of some medications including anti-compulsive drugs such as Prozac. None of these treatments has much of a success rate.

GUIDELINES TO HELP YOU DETERMINE FOR YOURSELF HOW BIG A PROBLEM A GUY'S KINKINESS REALLY IS

If you were to meet and be attracted to a man who has paraphilic interests, here are some questions to think about before forming a long-term attachment.

Is the behavior illegal? Remember, anything that is illegal might also be putting you at risk in a variety of ways. If he gets arrested, for example, and you have a job that requires a squeaky clean reputation, you may have work problems by virtue of your connection. You may also have financial problems that arise from legal bills.

Is the behavior maladaptive? In psychology we use the term maladaptive to describe behavior that is counterproductive. Counterproductive or maladaptive behavior works against the person's goals and deepest-held beliefs.

Is the behavior compulsive or addictive? Can the individual stop doing what he is doing or is he so compulsive about it that he is prepared to risk everything in order to continue doing it? If the paraphilia becomes like a drug and the person engaging in it starts behaving like an addict, it can create problems in your relationship similar to those caused by any addiction.

Does the behavior cause him personal unhappiness? Is the person engaging in the paraphilias in an almost constant state of conflict or despair caused by his paraphilic interests? Is he, for example, always worried about his secret being exposed or discovered? This level of distress is going to cause depression and anxiety and have an impact on every area of his life.

Is he engaging in consensual or nonconsensual activities? This is a major question. From my point of view, there is a major difference between a voyeur who occasionally visits a fetish sex club in order to watch people have sex and somebody who is chasing through backyards trying to peer in at strangers. I believe that all nonconsensual activities are potentially scary and should raise huge red flags!

WHAT ABOUT YOU AND YOUR ATTITUDE TOWARD SEX?

If you are attracted to a man with kinky sexual interests, you have to decide for yourself whether you will be comfortable and happy in this situation. Here are some things to consider.

Do you have a predominantly romantic view of sex? There is nothing wrong with viewing sex only as an extension of love and romance. Millions of women feel this way. However, if you have this point of view, it is highly unlikely that you are going to be happy with someone who is into experimentation and unusual behaviors. Think about it: You will be wanting to make eye contact and say, "I love you." He will be wanting you to stand over him with a riding crop and say things like "Bad boy. Down on your knees."

Do you feel as though you love him so much that you are willing to do anything for him, up to and including having sex in front of strangers? Wrong thinking! There is probably no single worse reason for getting involved with kinky sex than to try to to please a partner. It's a recipe for disaster and the chances are good that you will ultimately end up feeling perfectly horrible about the experience.

Are you curious and experimental about sex? If this is the case, you might be happy working out a sexual relationship with a kinky guy. Many women are. Also keep in mind that kinky men are often very enthusiastic about sex, and enthusiasm counts for a lot in my book.

SOME FINAL THOUGHTS

If you decide you want to experiment, my suggestion would be that you do it slowly and in a controlled environment. Don't jump in too quickly and get in over your head. You might want to experiment, for example, with something mildly kinky and see if you like it. You could try a little mild bondage, such as an easily undone scarf tying one hand to the bed or blindfolds during sex. Many couples find a way to incorporate one person's kinkiness into the relationship in an acceptable and legal way. If he's into voyeurism, for example, he peeks into his own bedroom window while his wife is undressing.

Also keep in mind that the more turned on you are, the more likely you might be to consent to something that's a little bit kinky. If you weren't turned on, you might think about a particular behavior and say, "Yuck!" But if you are really turned on, with the hormones flowing, it might be a whole different thing.

I guess the bottom line is that many guys with kinky interests are reasonably harmless and not dangerous, but you have to be comfortable with their dynamic. If, for example, you're with a guy with masochistic tendencies, and you are uncomfortable telling people what to do, particularly in bed, it's not going to work out. If you really like him, before you make any final decisions, educate yourself about what he's saying. Read material about different fetishes and what's involved. It's a whole other world out there. If you're with a kinky guy, you need to have some serious discussions so that you are both clear about what you will and won't do.

9

Getting Real About Illness, Meds, Drugs, and Booze

What happens with his body is going to have everything to do with what is happening in your bed. Take Brenda, for example: She has been married to her husband, Arthur, for thirty-five years. In those years, Brenda, Arthur, and the relationship have been through so many changes that it's hard for her even to recall some of the things that happened to them. They met right after college, and the attraction between them was instant and very strong. Back then, they would have round-the-clock sex, and it was great. Brenda still remembers the days when they were glued together; she had what appeared to be a permanent rash on her face and neck from his beard, and a chronic ache in her back and legs from having spent hours in various sexual positions. But life changed: Arthur got a job with long hours and a long commute; and their three daughters were born. That altered their sex life a lot. Then Arthur hurt his shoulder playing tennis and his knee playing golf and required surgery on both body parts. Between the two recuperations (they could only have sex with Brenda on top) and the pain medications (they got in the way of his erections), their sex life changed even more. Once their daughters were at college and out of the house, Sunday morning sex became a big treat, but Arthur developed diabetes and started having serious problems in bed. Brenda thought that sex would become nothing more than a memory, but then Arthur's doctor suggested that he try a performance enhancement medication. Well, Arthur is back and, in some ways, better than ever, except when his arthritic knee acts up.

A true fact of life: If the man in your bed develops an illness, starts taking medication, doing drugs, or indulges in heavy drinking, it is going to affect your sex life. Here are some of the things you need to know.

ILLNESS, MEDICAL CONDITIONS, AND SEX

Even something as simple as a cold can make any of us feel as though we don't want to have sex. I know I've said this before, but it's important enough to say again: If a guy starts experiencing sexual difficulties, the first thing he needs to do is get a complete medical workup. There are a variety of ailments and conditions that can have an impact on a guy's sexuality. These include:

Diabetes

This disease sometimes causes erection problems because it affects the nerves that activate blood flow to the penis. Unfortunately, this can happen to younger men as well as older men. I've known guys with diabetes who were able to have erections and experience all the sensations of orgasms, but who were no longer able to ejaculate. Some men with diabetes have opted for penile implants. In my personal experience, the men most likely to experience diabetes-related erection problems are men who are moderately to severely overweight.

Cardiovascular disease

For a guy to get an erection, he needs unimpaired blood flow. When a man starts experiencing difficulties getting or maintaining an erection, cardiovascular problems like arteriosclerosis and high blood pressure could be a contributing factor. This is more common as a man ages.

Prostate problems

With the exception of prostatitis, which can happen at any age, prostate problems are much more common in older men. Benign prostatic enlargement, for example, can have a negative impact on erections and ejaculations, as well as urination. Guys who develop prostatic cancer frequently receive treatments that affect erections. The complete radical surgical removal of the prostate, for example, can result in an inability to have an erection. Some men in this position opt for a penile implant. These guys can still have an orgasm even though they can't ejaculate. The good news is that some surgeons here and in Europe specialize in nerve-sparing surgery in order to help make it possible for men to continue to have erections. One of my clients had this kind of surgery in Europe, and I know that he was able to get a normal erection after having his prostate removed.

I recently read some material that indicates that many men are now being advised to follow a "use it or lose it" philosophy after prostate surgery. They are being given nightly doses of Viagra for several months following the operation. This is to encourage nighttime erections. Some men are also being given erection-enhancing injections for several weeks after their operations. These men are encouraged to masturbate as soon as they feel they can and to attempt sexual intercourse as soon as possible. After many of the various treatments such as radioactive seeds, men can typically still get erections, particularly if they decide to use erection-enhancing medications.

Prostatitis, which has nothing to do with prostate cancer, is an inflammation of the prostate gland. There are three types of prostatitis: acute, chronic, and noninfectious. The symptoms depend upon the type. Symptoms of acute prostatitis, for example, may include fever, chills, and pain, while the symptoms of chronic prostatitis can be almost nonexistent. All types of prostatitis require medical treatment. Prostatitis can sometimes be caused by an STD such as gonorrhea or chlamydia. If your partner develops prostatitis, it's probably a good idea to make sure that he is tested for these possibilities, and, if necessary, you should both be treated. In fact, when a man develops bacterial prostatitis, some doctors believe that both partners should be treated with an antibiotic. If the man in your life is diagnosed with prostatitis, you need to do your research about this and discuss it with your doctor.

Testicular cancer

Testicular cancer is more common among young men. It's very curable, particularly with early detection. More than one man has gone for early treatment because his girlfriend or wife, who may be more up close and personal with his testicles than he is, has said something along the lines of "Your balls look (or feel) a little funny—not funny, ha-ha, but funny, strange." Testicular cancer can also have an impact on sexual function. The symptoms of testicular cancer include:

- A lump or hardening in a testicle
- Pain or tenderness
- Fluid buildup in the scrotum
- An increase or decrease in the size of either testicle
- Blood in the semen

So if you feel a lump when you are fondling a guy's testicles or notice fluid buildup in his testicles or blood in his semen, tell him immediately so he can get to a doctor—the sooner the better. After having a testicle removed, a man can still have sex, but he might need testosterone replacement therapy.

Obesity

A guy's weight is going to make a difference in how he makes love. I have personally had sex with men who weighed in the four-hundred- to five-hundred-pound range (I'm not kidding), so I know that it is possible. I had a client who weighed around five hundred pounds, and, believe it or not, he was great in bed. Just don't ever let a heavyweight guy get on top! It's downright dangerous. When you're on top (which, I repeat, is where you have to be), it's sometimes kind of like having sex with a piece of furniture.

Sports injuries/mobility problems

Even young men can have issues such as sports injuries. Knee injuries can make sex very difficult. You usually have to use the female superior position. I know at least one guy who got in a cycling accident and dislocated his shoulder. Until it was fixed, he could also only use the female superior position. Arthritis is also challenging for your sex life. I find the side to side position works best under those conditions.

Concealed or hidden penis

This is an interesting condition in which a man gets fat and the fatty pad of his pubic mound engulfs the penile shaft, giving him the appearance of having a "hole" there rather than a penis. It only comes out when it's erect. Solutions usually include weight loss. There is also a surgery that can help correct this. I have seen several cases of hidden penis; the first time you see it, it freaks you out. For a minute, I really thought there was nothing there!

Peyronie's disease

You sometimes hear people joking about one guy or another who has an erection that curves or bends. Well, it's called Peyronie's disease, and it's no joke. Nobody can say definitively what causes Peyronie's disease, but it is sometimes associated with an injury caused by sex that is a little too enthusiastic. Sometimes it appears to develop almost overnight. At other times, however, the disease takes a slower course. The disease begins as a localized inflammation. In some mild cases, this inflammation resolves itself. In others, it goes on to form a hardened plaque or lump that makes the penis curve when there is an erection. Peyronie's disease can cause painful erections, particularly in the early stages. There are a variety of treatments, and these are most effective in the early stages. In short, if you and the man in your bed enjoy an exuberant night of lovemaking in which he seems to be pounding a little hard and in the next few days or weeks his erection becomes painful or shows any curvature, he needs to get to a doctor pronto.

Priapism

Anyone who has watched television advertisements for drugs for erectile dysfunction has probably noticed a sentence that reads something like this: "Consult a doctor if you have an erection that lasts longer than four hours." *Priapism* is the medical term used to describe a guy's erection when it won't go down, even though he is no longer being stimulated. Priapism is considered a medical emergency, and needs immediate treatment. Simply running it under a cold shower won't fix it! Priapism is sometimes associated with some underlying vascular or neurological conditions. It is also associated with alcohol or recreational drugs such as cocaine or amphetamine. It can also be connected to some prescription medications. Untreated priapism can have consequences and might involve serious and even permanent damage to the penis itself.

In short, if it doesn't go down, he needs to get to an emergency room!

Phimosis

This is a condition in which the foreskin of the uncircumsized penis is too tight, constricting the penis and often preventing an erection. Phimosis is sometimes seen in newborns, when it is known as infantile or congenital phimosis. When it develops in older males, it is known as acquired phimosis. It requires medical treatment such as stretching, medication, or sometimes circumcision.

PRESCRIPTION MEDICATION

Doesn't it sometimes seem as though everybody is on some kind of prescription medication? Whatever you have, there is a pill that might help. Men and women of all ages are on medication. ADD, ADHD, elevated blood pressure, depression, and anxiety are but a few of the more common conditions that are regularly treated with prescription medication. As wonderful and necessary as these medications can be, they can also have sexual side effects. For men, some of them reduce desire and an interest in sex; others interfere with erections; still others make it more difficult to have an orgasm and ejaculate. For some men, a few of these meds may even increase sexual activity.

If the guy in your life is taking any medication, you need to know that doctors are frequently reluctant to warn patients about sexual side effects. The concern is that if they mention it, the patient might have a psychological reaction and begin to anticipate, fear, or even imagine that the problem exists. Nonetheless, an extraordinarily large percentage of sexual difficulties can be directly traced to the use of medication.

Prescription drugs that may contribute to sexual issues include:

Blood pressure medications (including beta blockers and frequently prescribed diuretics such as hydrochlorothiazide)
Antidepressants such as selective serotonin reuptake inhibitors (SSRIs include Prozac, Zoloft, and Paxil) or MAO inhibitors (like Nardil, Parnate, and Marplan)
Medications for ADD and ADHD such as Adderall and Strattera
Cholesterol-lowering medications, including statins such as Lipitor

Remember that not everybody responds to medication in the same way, but if the guy in your life is taking any form of medication and starts having sexual issues, a call to the doctor or the pharmacy is in order. You should also know that many of these medications can be tweaked so that the difficulties are reduced or even disappear. Sometimes a substitute medication can be found or an additional one can be added to the mix. The message here is to make sure that nobody gives up on a drug that is helping without discussing it with a physician and finding equally effective treatment.

SEX AND BOOZE

I don't think anyone can talk about sexual activity in this day and age without a discussion of drinking and the sexual experience. Many women tell me that the first time they had sex, they were drinking. Other women have told me that they have rarely had sex when they were stone-cold sober. Let's be honest: Liquor, like some drugs, loosens inhibitions, increases desire, and can heighten the sexual experience, particularly when you are young and still have a healthy liver. I wouldn't be totally honest, however, if I didn't also tell you that alcohol ultimately has a very negative impact on sexuality. Nonetheless, if you are a sexually active woman who is attending parties or hanging out in clubs, it stands to reason that you are going to be meeting many men who can easily be described as having substance abuse issues. Sexy young guys with a buzz from alcohol are ubiquitous in these places. Many of the boozy guys you will meet are going to go home and sober up. Others are going to be going out and doing just as much drinking the next night and the next night and the next night. Before you get seriously involved with a guy, it is a good idea to get a clear handle on exactly how much he drinks and whether or not he can stop. It seems bizarre that so many of the women who hook up with guys with serious drug or alcohol problems say they didn't recognize either the problem or its severity until they were deeply involved.

Currently, Heather, for example, goes to at least three Al-Anon meetings a week trying to find better ways of handling her relationship with her husband, Matthew. When Heather first started sleeping with Matthew, they were both in their early twenties. They met at a party where they were both a little high. The sex was explosive, romantic, and raunchy—everything that great sex is supposed to be. That was then—eight years ago. This is now, and it's a whole new ball game. When they got married, Heather knew that Matthew drank a little bit more than he should, but so did she. So, by the way, did most of Matthew's friends. They were part of a crowd of successful men and women who liked to party. Heather and Matthew were young and in love and preparing for a fabulous future, and fun and frolic were part of what they expected. Then Heather got pregnant, and that changed everything. She got scared and immediately stopped drinking because she didn't want to do anything that might harm the pregnancy. Heather is now the sober mother of beautiful four-year-old twin girls. She can't run around with Matthew after work every night because she has two children in pre-K, and she wants to be home with her daughters. She has changed, but Matthew hasn't changed with her. Now a sober Heather cannot believe that she is married to a guy who is unquestionably an alcoholic. Heather still loves Matthew, but she hates the fact that he is more interested in getting a buzz than he is in talking about whether they should move to a better school district. These days, when they have sex, she is usually sober, while Matthew is still high. Heather finds it difficult to find the words that will sufficiently explain how boring sex can be under these conditions.

I know something about what Heather is feeling. About twenty years ago, I started a sexual relationship with a very attractive man.

At first, he was a great and very romantic lover. Over the years, in addition to drinking more and more, he started using pot very heavily. Pretty soon, his sexual abilities started to go into the toilet, and I don't mean to suggest that his sexual functioning was the only area of his life that deteriorated. He couldn't keep a job and his life generally fell apart. Despite his problems, we remained friends for almost seventeen years, but his issues finally were more than he or anyone else could handle. Now, I was not married to him, nor was he even my primary relationship. Nonetheless, I remember my anxiety and frustration as I tried to think of things that might disrupt his downward spiral, but nothing helped, and he is now dead.

Estimates on the number of people with alcohol dependency vary greatly. Here in the United States it's estimated to be anywhere from five to ten percent of the population, or even higher. All I can say with any certainty is that if you are a sexually active woman, there is a great likelihood that you will meet a fair number of men who drink regularly. Some of these men will make a concerted effort, often joining AA, and manage to stop drinking; some of these men will turn forty or thereabouts and spontaneously stop or cut back on their drinking; and some of these men will evolve into major league substance abusers. I don't know how to tell for sure which guy will go in which direction, and I don't think anyone else can either.

Here is some of what I do know. Heavy drinkers can be very attractive and appealing. For one thing, some guys who are drunk become wildly romantic. They can say everything you want to hear and do everything you want them to do. There is a country and western song about a guy who "marries a waitress." The next day he has a major predicament because he doesn't know her name. I know a woman who is married to a man who has been married five times. He says the first four don't count because he was "drunk as a skunk." My message in this is that if you meet a man who is drink-

ing and he sweeps you off your feet saying wonderful things, don't be surprised if he doesn't remember anything that he said and did and, even worse, doesn't want to be reminded. In fact, you could establish a relationship and that could be a continuing pattern: When he is drinking, he will send e-mails and make phone calls, telling you how much he loves you. When he is sober, he is like a different guy. In fact, sober, he could seem boring and much less interesting than he did when he was drunk.

There are a couple of other things you need to keep in mind about heavy drinkers. They don't always appear or act drunk to you. This is particularly true if the guy is younger and still hasn't done serious damage to his liver or his brain. Also, some guys who are compulsive drinkers are also compulsive sexually. More than one woman has fallen in love with a man who can best be described as a womanizer with a drinking problem.

Many heavy drinkers pride themselves on their sexual prowess, and to be perfectly honest, it can actually be true when they are still young. But over time, alcohol will damage the central nervous system and destroy brain cells. From their extensive research, Masters and Johnson believed alcohol led to male impotence. Anecdotally, if yo talk to hundreds of men and women as I have, you will come to same conclusion. Most sophisticated and sexually experienced wo know what it is like to be with a man whose liquor consumptic left him without an erection or the ability to ejaculate. At first temporary, but over time, it can become a chronic situation.

RECREATIONAL DRUGS

Drugs are considered a "social trap"—an activity th ing in the short term, but has potentially harmful

consequences in the long term. In fact, all recreational drugs that I am aware of have harmful sexual consequences in the long term. I try to tell my students this, but I'm not sure that they are paying attention. Statistically, one of the main arguments against recreational drugs is that these substances put you at a huge risk of catching an STD because drug use frequently accompanies reckless behavior and poor judgment. I certainly remember what it is to be young and high, and it would be completely hypocritical of me to be judgmental about people who use recreational drugs. Having said that, I would also like to add that times have changed since I was in my twenties: The kinds and quality of drugs that are around these days are substantially different. For the most part, people in my generation were exposed to a little bit of weak pot, which did often heighten sexual desire, along with giving you the munchies. From what I can see, college kids today are exposed to a wide compendium of strong and sometimes even lethal recreational drugs. Even the marijuana tends to be stronger.

The other risk involved with recreational drug use, of course, is that they are illegal. If you are joining the guy in your life in his quest for drugs, you run the risk of being on the more dangerous side of the law. This will cost you time as well as money. Although there is certainly a lot of drama involved in being in a relationship with a drug user, most of the time it is no fun. The question of sexual dysfunction and whether or not he can "get it up" will quickly become the least of your problems. Cheryl, for example, lives with a guy who does a lot of drugs. Donald has a staid middle-class job and goes months without doing any drugs—and then out of the blue, when she least expects it, he goes MIA on her. Then there is usually a period of a week or two when her only contact with him is when he calls in the middle of the night from his cell phone. "I love you baby," he slurs before hanging up. While he is

"out," Cheryl has to field other calls as well. His mother, his ex-wife, his son, his boss, and his sister all phone regularly. Sometimes Cheryl also gets calls from his dealer. Cheryl never knows for sure whether Donald is alive, dead, in jail, or in a hospital. After one of his outings, he returned without his car. Cheryl was never able to figure out what happened to it. Was it wrecked? Was it stolen? Did he sell it to buy more drugs? When Donald reappears, smelly and needing a shave, he sometimes checks into rehab for a few days, but more often he just comes home. Donald is very good at what he does for a living, which is why he manages to find work, but even so, he tends to burn through his jobs. He also goes through a lot of money. One of his little excursions into the drug world will typically cost up to ten or twenty thousand dollars. He does not do injectable drugs, but nonetheless it occurs to Cheryl that he might end up having sex with somebody who does and might thus increase his risk for getting a serious STD, like HIV. She doesn't worry about it all that much, however. She says, "When he is doing drugs, his interest in sex is pretty much nonexistent. Besides, we don't really have sex anymore either." Cheryl is trying to end the relationship, but she has known Donald for a long time, and it's very difficult.

Here are some of the most common recreational drugs along with sexual side effects.

Nicotine

Yes, smoking is really bad for a guy's sexual health. It constricts the small blood vessels, especially in the face, hands, and genitals. Consequently, nicotine is bad for erections. In other words, if you fall for a chain smoker when he is still young, there is a good chance that he will develop problems with his erection later in life.

Marijuana

In the short term, smoking pot focuses the senses and can make the experience much more intense and sensual—so long as it's not so strong that it puts you to sleep. In the long term, I hate to be the one to tell you this, but unfortunately, marijuana can cause a lowered sperm count and a lowered sex drive. Some men who smoke a lot of pot also tend to lose the motivation to have sex. Another side effect of long-term use for men can be male breast development.

Cocaine

In the short term, cocaine can make a guy seem hypersexual and help him have a longer-lasting erection. With regular long-term use, however, cocaine has been known to lower desire and can cause erection problems. Women who sleep with guys who use a lot of cocaine tend to have war stories to tell about men with faltering erections.

Heroin and other opiates

These tend to lower desire. Users are already high and frequently lose interest in having sex. You don't need me to tell you that having sex with somebody who is doing any injectable drugs will put you at a much, much higher risk of contracting HIV, along with other STDs.

Ecstasy

This used to be thought of as the "love drug" because it was supposed to put you in touch with your inner feelings (but what if your inner feelings are homicidal rage?). The primary ingredient in ecstacy is MDMA (methylenedioxymethamphetamine). This includes the stimulant properties of methamphetamine (similar to the street drug known as crystal meth) along with hallucinogenics. There are so many problems associated with ecstacy, or "e" as it is sometimes called, that it's difficult to list them. One of the major ones, however, is that there is no quality control of individual pills and there are a variety of substances that could be included, some of which are deadly. For some people, there is a short-term euphoria associated with ecstacy that may heighten sensuality. Long term, it can lead to feelings of depression and loss of desire.

Methamphetamine

Methamphetamine, which is also known as "meth" or "crystal meth," can be injected, snorted, or smoked, and it is a very dangerous drug. I have a friend—let's call him Samuel—who I've known for years. When I first met him, he was very interested in sex and had a variety of female friends. Then several years ago he started using methamphetamine, heavily. He was snorting it, not injecting it. After about a year of doing this, he reached the point where he couldn't even get an erection at all and wasn't interested in sex anyway. Currently, he's definitely in bad shape: His physical and mental health have both deteriorated. He has a wide variety of physical problems and has become so paranoid that he is scary. I still talk to him every now and then. When I do, I spend most of the time trying to convince him to get some help with his health.

Methamphetamine tends to lower inhibitions and is also one of those drugs that is associated with extremely risky sexual behavior. Some users report that meth increases their sex drive and makes them crave sex. They also say that they are able to have sex for longer periods of time. However, as much as they may desire sex, they are frequently unable to ejaculate or have orgasms.

A SPECIAL WARNING TO WOMEN

If you are in a relationship with an alcoholic or drug user, you probably don't need me to tell you of the challenges you face, ranging from avoiding the role of the enabler to resisting being drawn into his world. Many women have found that organizations such as Al-Anon have helped them set boundaries and find realistic ways of dealing with their relationships.

10

Good and Great Lovers: What They Do and Don't Do

What makes a lover good? What makes him great? Is there any way you can know ahead of time how a guy is going to behave in bed? My answer to that question is always "Probably not." Good and even great lovers, of whom I've had more than my share, come in all different sizes and shapes. You can't tell by looking at a guy, or even watching him move, what he is going to be like in bed. You can't tell by the width of his shoulders, the size of his hands, or how much hair he has or doesn't have on his head. The best lover in your neighborhood could be the skinny, short guy you see hunched over his coffee at the Starbucks every morning reading the *Wall Street Journal.* He could even be the heavyset guy you see at the supermarket trying to keep track of three kids while he buys breakfast cereal. In other words, great lovers don't necessarily work out and they don't always look so hot either. Conversely, the cutest, sexiest-looking guy you know with the best toned butt could be really clueless when it comes to lovemaking.

By now, you've probably figured out that a certain amount of my sexual experience has been skewed toward dealing with guys with problems, but that's not how I see my sex life in retrospect. In fact, I've had many, many more good sexual experiences than bad ones. There is no comparison, and I can literally count the bad

experiences on one hand. That does not mean that I haven't had my
share of clueless lovers, and I know that you too will probably meet
some men who are completely out to lunch when it come to sex and
how to please a woman. However, I also know that you will meet
men who are so good in bed that they will leave you with your
knees shaking and your eyes rolling back in your head.

Sometimes, of course, the sex is particularly memorable because it's
an attractive new guy, and the sex is taking place in unique or exciting
circumstances. I remember years ago lying by myself on a small beach
in Lahaina, Maui. I was reading a book and getting ready to go back
to my hotel room. It was late afternoon, maybe five o'clock. A man
walked toward me carrying a bag. He was wearing sunglasses. He
stopped and looked at me and took off the sunglasses. He had really
unusual blue eyes. He said, "I just bought a six pack of beer at the liquor store. Would you like to help me drink it?" I was about to say no,
but he was kind of good-looking, about my age, and so I said, "Why
not?" Remember, I was on vacation. So we drank the beer and he was
really nice and funny and we were both really attracted to each other.
There were several boats moored offshore there, and he suggested we
go to his friend's boat. The tide was so low that we could wade there.
So we waded out to the boat, which was not large, but had a lot of
cushions, and we had sex. It was one of those "I've just been out in the
sun all day so I'm really horny" sessions. He told me he was the captain
of a dive boat and asked if he could see me the next day. But I was leaving the next day! I liked him so much I made plans to go back on
spring break to stay with him for ten days. We had sex everywhere: on
the beach, on rocks, on the side of a volcano. Sexually, he was really
hot and had a very unusual penis. He claimed it was a circumcision accident, but his penis had these "belt loops" on it—two strands of tissue
that connected the head to the shaft. I have some photographs of it
somewhere with flowers stuck through the belt loops. (Yes, *Lady*

Chatterley's Lover was an early influence on my life.) I gave him oral sex while perched on a rock just below a lookout where tourists were taking pictures of whales. He had the most unusual tasting semen—it tasted like salt water—no surprise. We continued our relationship off and on for close to sixteen years. We used to joke about the fact that every time we saw each other, we both had at least one orgasm. From a technical standpoint he was a very sensuous and lusty guy who had all the qualities that make for a good lover. When I think about the sex itself, however, it was somewhat predictable, but in a very good way. Part of the reason why it felt so special and great had to do with the context and the setting. The same ho-hum sex acts you enjoy with your husband in your bedroom after watching the nightly news would have a different impact if they took place on the side of a volcano, as much of our sex did.

Having said that, let's talk a bit about what makes a guy good (or even great) in bed.

GOOD LOVERS ARE PASSIONATE

Whether you call it enthusiasm, passion, desire, lust, or just plain old-fashioned horniness, there is nothing more exciting, or more of a turn-on, than a guy who has a way of letting you feel his sexual energy. Don't we all agree that passion is what makes sex sexy? The thing is, though, that guys have different ways of expressing intensity and sexual desire: Some do it with words, some do it with their eyes, and some do it with very specific body language. A guy doesn't have to move like Elvis Presley to convey sexual energy. I remember one man I knew who bit one corner of his bottom lip when he was turned on. I know it sounds weird, but you had to be there to appreciate what that little movement came to express to me.

Do you remember the first time you slow-danced with a guy and you felt his penis becoming erect? Sarah does. She says, "It was a senior high school dance, and a boy I hardly knew asked me to dance. We were slow dancing and I couldn't help but notice that he was hard. I must have pulled away a little, because he said, "Sorry, I can't help it. It's the way you make me feel." He managed to control himself, but his voice said it all. We dated for that whole summer before college, and he always made it clear that he thought I was totally sexy and desirable. It's been twenty years, but I still remember that dance and how weak-kneed it made me feel."

Annie remembers an affair she had with a coworker that began when they were out of town together on business. She says, "We were staying in the same motel, in different rooms, of course, and we went out for dinner at the restaurant that was connected to the motel. There had always been a little flirtation between the two of us and during dinner it became apparent that it was much more than a little flirtation. We started dinner sitting in a booth opposite each other and by the time we were finished, he had moved over to my side. He was kissing my neck, and his hand was between my legs. He put my hand on his crotch, and I didn't stop anything he was doing. Finally, he said, 'Let's get out of here,' and motioned to the waiter so he could pay the bill.

"To get back to the motel itself, you were supposed to walk around the restaurant on a path, but there was a more direct route if you were prepared to jump over a split rail fence. That's what he did. He said, 'I don't think I can wait to take your clothes off,' and he jumped over the fence. Then he reached over and picked me up and over the fence as well. It was a cold, crisp winter night with snow on the ground. The moon was full and there were stars in the sky. I still remember the crunchy sound my feet made in the snow when he put me down. We ran to my motel room. He was such a passionate guy!"

You will note that these stories are all about those moments leading up to actual sex, and it's interesting how many women remember more about the passion involved in the lead-up to sex than they do about the sex itself. But how a guy shows his sexual energy once you are actually making love is equally important. Once they get into bed, I divide men into three passion categories. As you can see, I'm a little like Goldilocks.

1. Too physically intense

Yes, this guy has passion, but the only way he knows how to show it is by excessive physical activity. He is pretty clueless when it comes to understanding sexual energy or women's bodies. He behaves as if he has to carry the whole show and believes he should be moving or doing something the whole time. Typically this man is used to being rough with his own penis. That's what he likes, and he thinks he should touch women the same way. He doesn't know how to slow down, he has never explored the many levels of physical intimacy, and he doesn't know how to convey any emotion except excessive urgency. He's the Energizer bunny, and he's on top of you! Eek! After you've had sex with one of these guys, you feel like you just went ten rounds with Hulk Hogan. It's like having sex with a jackhammer. His whole approach conveys the sense that you don't really matter; he could be having sex with anyone.

2. Too mellow

This guy may be feeling all kinds of things, but he isn't showing any of it. He's not physically active enough and appears clueless about communicating his intensity. It's as if he doesn't know what to do. He acts almost fearful, as if too much movement or activity would make you wince. Even worse, he can appear almost bored or disinterested. He rarely says anything, and when he does it's usually something along the lines of "Can you move your leg to the right?" His whole approach conveys the sense that he doesn't even know that he is having sex, let alone who he is having it with.

3. Just right

The guy who knows how to convey passion and sexual energy in bed understands nuance and intensity. He knows when to move quickly and when to slow down and take his time. He always appears turned on specifically by you, and even if he is sometimes acting a little bit, so what. Most important, he knows how to make you feel that you matter. He desires you, and he wants to please you. You can feel his sexual energy by what he says and what he does. You feel as though it's something about you that's inspiring him, and it's a great feeling.

GOOD LOVERS ARE SPONTANEOUS AND ABLE TO HAVE FUN WITH SEX

Belinda's boyfriend Ed is a balding medical doctor with the beginning of a paunch. Although he is only in his early thirties, he appears years older. Everything about him screams out "respectable and responsible"—everything, that is, except his approach to sex. As far as sex is concerned, Belinda says that Ed is a "wild man" and she loves it. Belinda describes Ed as the "King of Spontaneous Sex." She says, "Sex with him is exciting because you never know when he is going to get interested. He can get so turned on when we are at the movies that he doesn't want to wait until the end of the movie. Once, we were at a fancy wedding about fifteen miles from where we live.

Instead of going home, he turned into a motel and we pretended it was prom night, and we were high school kids having sex for the first time. He undressed me slowly as if he had never done it before. It was so much fun—also very sexy. Ed laughs and says he has a preoccupation with unplanned sex, but I actually think he fantasizes about and plans at least some of our more 'spontaneous' moments. It doesn't matter because I really love that he has a creative attitude toward sex. I especially love that he makes me feel so desirable."

A great lover is able to be spontaneous in a way that turns you on. He seems to know when you are feeling sexual. A clueless lover, on the other hand, seems to have an unerring instinct for those moments when spontaneous sex is the last thing on your mind and far from fun. A clueless lover, for example, is demanding without making sure that you share his mood. He might decide that he is ready for spontaneous sex just as you are basting the Thanksgiving turkey and putting the finishing touches on the dinner you are preparing for your whole family, who are due to arrive in ten minutes. If you stop doing what you are doing, the corn soufflé will fall, the pie will burn along with the stuffing, and you will be serving dinner to your mother and father in your underwear.

A great lover, on the other hand, seems able to know instinctively when your hormones are flowing—even when you don't know it yourself. Once, many years ago, I was involved with one of my coworkers, and I came to work early in the morning. He was the only other person there. I remember looking down at my pantyhose and saying, "Oh, damn! I've got a run in my pantyhose." He said, "What are you going to do with them?" I said, "Throw them in the trash." He said, "I have a better idea" and gave me one of those looks that romance writers describe as smoldering. Now remember, this was a sex clinic, so we definitely had beds there. So we went into one of the rooms, and he proceeded to take the pantyhose off me with his teeth. Now, if I wasn't in the mood or into the guy, this might not have been a turn-on, but I was. By the time we were finished, my pantyhose was hanging in rags around us.

A spontaneous, good lover seems able to pick the unusual spots and moments in a way that will work. The clueless lover does exactly the opposite. I remember one unfortunate experience with a guy who convinced me to go into an idyllic-looking cow pasture on a summer evening. It was a mistake I'm not likely to repeat again.

GOOD LOVERS HAVE OPTIONS

My friend Heidi says one of the best lovers she ever knew was Jonathan, a man who had studied several Asian philosophies. He was skilled at various meditation techniques, tai chi, and yoga. Like many men who are students of Eastern philosophies, he had learned how to use what he knew to sexual advantage. Jonathan's erection was totally reliable. In fact, Jonathan seemed to have complete control of both his erections and his ejaculations. Jonathan, who was in his fifties when Heidi met him, had no problem with doing quickies, but he also had no problem with incredibly long and extended periods of lovemaking devoted to pleasing Heidi. When Heidi asked Jonathan what gave him so much control, he said that his tai chi and meditation practice made it all possible. He said it also increased his pleasure.

Not all lovers are going to be as accomplished as Jonathan in terms of their ability to control their erections. Yet there is no question that some of the confidence that good lovers exude at least in part comes from their knowledge that they are in charge of their erections.

I remember one guy I had sex with a few years back. He was amazing. Almost as soon as we met, it was apparent that there was great chemistry. He invited me out for dinner the next night, and the sparks were igniting all over the place. He came back to my house and we had sex. And then we had sex again. And again! I had never been with anyone with a sexual appetite like this. He could literally have intercourse and ejaculate every half hour for about ten hours. After about the fifth or six round (I lost count), I remember saying to him, "Have any sexual researchers ever studied you? Because they definitely should!" Since then, I've certainly had lovers I've enjoyed and some I've been in love with, but I never met anybody who could equal him.

In addition to being fantastic from a mechanical standpoint, he was intelligent and funny. He also knew how to compliment a woman and kept up almost a nonstop conversation filled with verbal flattery. He was an ordinary-looking guy—certainly no movie star—and you wouldn't know by looking at him that he was great in bed.

GOOD LOVERS LIKE AND UNDERSTAND WOMEN'S BODIES

A good lover has taken the time to learn more about a woman's body. He has made a point of knowing as much as he can about female anatomy and physiology. He knows where everything is. He understands the various ways a woman can have an orgasm. He knows how sensitive the clitoris can be. Ditto a woman's breasts. He has taken the time to learn what's going on inside a woman's vagina. He knows that all women are a little bit different, and that just because he was able to bring his last girlfriend to orgasm by licking her big toe doesn't mean that it's going to work with anyone else. When a guy takes the time to figure out what he should be doing, it can have amazing results. My friend Joan said that when she was still in her twenties she had sex with an equally young guy. He was kind of a geeky math major who was also a virgin. Nonetheless, he was amazing. She couldn't help asking him, "How do you know so much about women's bodies and what to do?" His answer surprised her. He said, "I read a bunch of books."

I personally don't like it when guys pretend to be comfortable about women's bodies when they really are not. I always remember one clueless guy who said to me, "Do you have your period now?" "Yes," I replied. I was about to remark on how perceptive he was when he floored me with the next sentence: "So can we have anal sex instead?"

GOOD LOVERS KNOW HOW TO USE WORDS

Women are very in tune with wanting to hear nice, loving, sexy things while they make love. The best lovers know enough to say things like "I love the way your breasts feel in my hands." Or "I always get excited when I touch your skin." A simple "You're so beautiful" is never a bad thing to say. I have a friend who tells me that her boyfriend always admires her body when they are about to have sex. "Do you know," he asks her, "how many women in this world would do anything to have a body like yours?"

I remember one of the best sex talkers I ever knew. He had a constant narration going on—"this is great, this feels wonderful, your breasts are so beautiful." I admit it, I'm a sucker for that kind of thing. I always say, "I'm looking for a man with a large vocabulary, or if not that, then a big dictionary." He also said things that made me laugh. I remember cracking up when he said, "Whenever I look at your legs, my brain sends a message down to my balls that says, 'Start production!'" He would nuzzle into my boobs for about half an hour and then say, "I've always been a leg man."

A good lover is sensitive to the kinds of words his partner wants to hear. He doesn't start screaming things like "Do me good, you big, fat slut" in her ear unless he knows that she finds it exciting (which, by the way, she probably doesn't).

Great lovers also know how to ask questions: They know how to ask you where you want to be touched and what they can do to make sure you have an orgasm.

Good lovers also know how to use words to be directive without being demanding. I love men who are able to use their words in a sensual way to tell me what they want me to touch or do; conversely I hate it when men turn into demanding bedroom choreographers. My friend Anna remembers one clueless guy who always wanted his balls to be touched in a certain way during sex that was almost physically impossible to do. He would give the same kind of specific directions using the same kind of voice that he might use when telling a lost motorist how to get back on a highway, and he would get annoyed because her arms weren't long enough to do what he wanted. It was *so* not sexy!

GOOD LOVERS ARE CAREFUL

There are so many ways in which the best lovers are careful. Let's start with health concerns: There is no excuse for a man not being careful about issues of health or possible pregnancy. A good lover has current information about birth control and sexually transmitted diseases. He has latex condoms and expects to use them to help prevent sexually transmitted diseases. He is able to have an intelligent conversation about birth control, and he understands the method you are using and is cooperative.

No woman below a certain age can have sex without considering the possibility of pregnancy, and no woman of any age can have sex without thinking about protection against STDs. A good lover understands and appreciates his partner's concerns.

Good lovers are also careful about a wide variety of other things about which a woman might be concerned. I had a friend who met a guy at a party and went back to his apartment with him and spent the night. They saw each other about once a week for more than a month before she returned to *his* apartment. When they got to the bedroom, they sat on the side of the bed, and my friend couldn't help but notice several long blonde hairs on the pillow. They matched hers. She picked one up and dangled it in front of his face. "It's yours," the guy assured her. "I don't want you to think anyone else has been here since I met you." He was so clueless that he couldn't seem to understand that she was upset about the hair not because she was jealous, but because he had been sleeping on the same sheets for at least six weeks.

GOOD LOVERS ARE ROMANTIC

What woman doesn't appreciate a romantic lover? My friend Lynette says that recently she went to spend a weekend with her boyfriend Juan, who is currently working out of town and living in a hotel for several months. When she got to his hotel room, she discovered that he had filled the room with flowers, had champagne chilling in a bucket, and had replaced the bulbs in the hotel lamps with pink ones so it would look more romantic. Lynette was thrilled.

Patti says her boyfriend plans and arranges romantic picnics in all kinds of weather, and that it is always romantic. On cold winter evenings, they have picnic dinners in the living room in front of the fire. He also regularly lights candles all around the bathroom, and fills the tub with bubbles so that he and Patti can bathe together. She says, "I melt every time."

Jennifer remembers the Valentine's Day her husband came home with a gorgeous red lace bra (in her size), panties to match, and an incredibly beautiful red silk dress. He insisted she wear everything when they went out that evening. Then, in the restaurant, he kept telling her how much he was looking forward to removing them when they got home.

Some men know how to use food to set a romantic scene. I've had a couple of boyfriends who romanced me by cooking—often wonderful Italian meals. Years ago when I still worked for the post office, a coworker and I started a little flirtation. At the post office, you work weird, rotating days, but one week we happened to both have Saturday off. He asked me to go for a picnic with him to a beach in Palos Verdes. It was an unseasonably warm and gorgeous day in December. He said he would bring all the food, so I wasn't expecting much. We had to climb down a cliff to get to this secluded beach. I couldn't believe the food he brought—wonderful wine, chicken breasts, Brie, and all kinds of gourmet appetizers. We were totally alone on this secluded nude beach and, as you can imagine, one thing led to another. How did I let this guy slip away from me?

I have another friend who remembers the opposite kind of experience. A man she worked with suggested a picnic and also said he would bring everything. He took her to a lake that had been having a problem with algae. The water was totally receded and there were mounds of dead fish everywhere. For the food, he brought American cheese sandwiches on stale white bread and Diet Dr Pepper. Another friend of mine went home with a man who convinced her to come back to his house with him because he said he would light a fire in his fireplace and they could toast marshmallows. When he lit the fire, something was wrong with the flue and the room was immediately filled with dark smoke. This is the kind of thing that could happen to anyone, but what made this guy a failure in the romantic lover department was his refusal to acknowledge the smoke, which was making it almost impossible to breathe. "Let's have sex first," he insisted. "Then we can call the fire department."

Not every man is going to be totally romantic every time you make love. From my point of view, I don't even need romance every time. But there is no question that a romantic man makes a woman feel special. This helps her feel more responsive and trusting, which inevitably translates into much better sex.

GOOD LOVERS ARE CONFIDENT

Confidence is a large part of good lovemaking. Confident lovers know that they have the power to please a woman and it shows in everything they do in bed. They know that they know how to touch your body; they know that they know how to kiss; they know that they know how to bring you to orgasm. Confident guys are sure of who they are. This means that they are not afraid to show their vulnerabilities and their humanity.

I remember one guy I knew—let's call him Marc. Marc was very experienced and had been to bed with hundreds of women. He always knew exactly where to touch me and when. He was sure enough of himself that he wasn't embarrassed about admitting it when he felt tired. I remember times when we had sex once and then started again, and he needed more of a refractory period before he could have another orgasm. He knew how to say, "Let's rest and finish up later. I need a break here."

A confident lover is able to play your body like an instrument; he gives you the sense that you are in good hands. The other thing about a confident lover, like a confident driver, is that he isn't afraid to ask for directions. "Do you want me to touch here? Or here? Or how about here?" As he is saying it, you know that he isn't lost, but that he always wants to take the more scenic route.

The opposite of confidence is the guy who starts bragging about how great he is, no matter what he is doing. I remember one clueless guy who said to me, "Hey baby, how do you like my big d***?" In fact, not only did he not have a big d***, he didn't even have an erection! What was he thinking?

GOOD LOVERS ARE ABLE TO FOCUS ON SEX WITHOUT DISTRACTIONS

When you are in bed with a man, you want him to be paying attention to you. I personally have been in bed with guys who seem to have sexual ADD. They have all kinds of other things going on—a television tuned to CNN, a radio set to NPR, a cell phone that rings frequently, a landline attached to an answering machine that can be heard picking up messages, and flickering computer monitors. As soon as sex is finished, they hop out of bed to play back messages or return calls. It's best to make love in a room with no distractions, no background news shows, and no phones.

GOOD LOVERS ARE GOOD LISTENERS

One of the best lovers I know is someone with whom I worked for many years. Jackson was a male sexual surrogate at the time; he worked successfully with dozens of women, many of whom were in sex therapy because they were fearful of men. Sometimes they would spend up to a year just talking before they felt comfortable about having any physical contact. Jackson was very sensitive to women, and he knew how to listen to what they were expressing with their words as well as their body language. He was a very special guy and a really great lover.

In the world of sexual relationships, there is no question that a really great lover pays attention to what his partner is telling him. Even more important, however, a really great lover wants to know and understand more about his partner. He is interested in her! So many women complain about men who never listen. Truly great lovers not only listen, they ask questions. They want you to tell them where to touch you and when to touch you. They want you to help them turn you on, so they pay attention to what you say.

GOOD LOVERS HAVE A PLEASURE- VERSUS PERFORMANCE-BASED ORIENTATION

I used to date this guy who was so focused on the idea of having multiple orgasms that it wasn't any fun to have sex with him. He was sort of grading himself on what he was doing the entire time we had sex. Many guys approach sex as though it's a task to be completed. They sort of close their eyes and do what they think should be done without savoring the moments. Sometimes these men always do everything in exactly the same way. This is the guy who always spends two and a half minutes kissing, then two and half minutes on oral sex, then two and a half minutes in the missionary position, then bingo, orgasm, which is the goal. It's exactly the same way every night. It's boring.

Really good lovers are guided more by what they are feeling at the moment. If the kissing is pleasurable, for example, they stay with it. Sex with these guys doesn't feel scripted, and it doesn't feel constrained by expectations or goals. They are able to explore and experiment with sex. If something doesn't work, like having sex on the kitchen counter surrounded by pots and pans, they are able to laugh and let it go. Sex is supposed to be fun, right!?

GOOD LOVERS ARE SENSUAL AND WANT TO KISS AND TOUCH EVERYWHERE

Slow, sensual kissing and touching of all the body parts is the perfect way to start making love. For example, I really enjoy it when a guy knows how to give a good massage. I have a friend who says that one of the best lovers she ever had was a guy who had problems with his erections. Nonetheless he made up for it by being an expert at sensual massage. He would light candles and begin on her back, slowly massaging her legs, buttocks, neck, head, and back before turning her over and massaging and kissing the front of her body. He would then finish up by performing oral sex on her—which brings us to one of the most important good lover requirements.

A GOOD LOVER LOVES TO DO ORAL SEX

As much as I love oral sex, I literally don't remember the first time I experienced a man performing oral. What I do know is that many very unlikely candidates are really great at oral. I remember this one guy, Victor, who was this scholarly looking man with big thick glasses. He would go down on me and keep his glasses on because he said he didn't want to miss anything. But his glasses would get all steamed up. The guy who is good at oral sex dives right in without being asked. He goes at it with gusto, but not hard enough so you want to back away. He uses a lot of tongue and really gets into what he's doing.

I know some people are into combining food and sex, but I'm not really a fan of emptying out the refrigerator. To me, eating whipped cream off genitals is a little like eating an ice cream cone and finding pubic hairs on it. I sometimes feel like I should get a tattoo on my stomach with an arrow pointing down that says "No food or drink allowed in this area."

I know that many people disagree with me on this, and if you like the whipped cream approach, then by all means go for it!

A WARNING ABOUT SOME OF THE GREAT LOVERS YOU MAY MEET

Before we finish up this chapter, I think we should acknowledge that just because he's good in bed doesn't mean that he's a good guy.

If you are like most women, it is entirely possible that some of the best lovers you will meet will be narcissistic performance artists who will wow you in bed, but who have the power to leave you scratching your head or clutching your heart. Take Ian, for example. He is without question the most amazing lover Sandi has ever known. He always knows exactly what to say; he always knows exactly what to do. Sex with him has variety, spice, and intensity. Sometimes they make love in the light and he looks deeply into her eyes as he encourages her pleasure; sometimes they make love in the shower or in the bath; sometimes he rolls over first thing in the morning and surprises her. Whether it's light or dark, day or night,

Ian always sounds passionate and enthusiastic. Sometimes he is tender and gentle; other times he is athletic and vigorous. He also has amazing control and can last forever. He is proficient at oral sex and he is a master of massage and passionate body kisses. Wow, he is just the best, and Sandi is totally into him and everything he does in bed. So what is the problem?

There was no problem until Sandi discovered that Ian was sleeping with two other women. She asks, "How can he have sex with me all weekend, tell me he loves me, and then two days later be doing the same thing with somebody else? Why does he want to do that?" Sandi needs to understand that Ian is a performance artist and a supreme narcissist. In Ian's self-centered world, Sandi barely exists. As far as he's concerned, she's interchangeable with dozens of other women. Yes, of course, he is attracted to her. And, yes, of course, he likes the fact that she likes him. He may even love her, as much as he is capable of love, but that doesn't mean that he is ever going to be honest, faithful, or genuinely committed.

One of the reasons these men are so good in bed is that they have had so much rehearsal time. So many women have had their hearts broken by men who fall into the Casanova tradition that I don't think we can talk about great lovers without acknowledging that they exist. These are men who are great in bed and hell in relationships. I have certainly fallen for a couple of these guys, as have most other women I know.

So can you have a sexual relationship with a narcissistic performance artist? Of course you can, and it might absolutely be the greatest sex of your life. You run into trouble when you take these men seriously or think about them as having the potential to be good life partners. Just remember to keep some self-protective emotional distance and maintain realistic expectations.

THE BOTTOM LINE

What makes you happiest in bed? Every woman remembers at least one guy who had a signature move that turned her to jelly, and every woman has her own checklist for what she considers great. If you really like a specific guy, all rules about what is or isn't good in bed go out the window. And let's not forget that the chemistry between you and a particular man may be so intense that everything he does seems great. Good sex is sex that feels good to you, and a great lover is a lover who pleases you!

11

Summing Up: The Sex Therapist's Best Advice

I don't mean to brag, but I really do know a great deal about sex. Over the years, I've worked with hundreds of men of all ages who had sexual issues and I've seen them evolve into good, and sometimes great, lovers. As you can imagine, I've learned a fair amount from all my sexual experiences. Here are some of the most important things I'd like to tell other women.

TRY TO GET PAST YOUR INHIBITIONS ABOUT TALKING TO MEN ABOUT SEX

As you can imagine, I've had more experience than most women in talking to men about what they do in bed. I will also admit that there is something in my personality that encourages people to talk about sex. I've always figured that it's because I have more of a masculine attitude about sexuality, but I've had complete strangers come up to me and start discussing sex in a fairly clinical way. I guess I enjoy talking about sex (which is a good thing considering my occupation). With most of the men I've known, once they learned about my professional background, they didn't want to talk about anything else. I'm embarrassed to admit that I knew one man for about ten years, sharing many conversations of an intimate nature, before I discovered that he was once a prisoner of war, and I only found that out by reading the newspaper.

Despite my personal experience, I know that talking to men about sex can be very challenging. Remember that some men are typically nervous about these conversations because they don't want to do or say anything that turns you off. They don't have the vocabulary or the experience, and they know it. There are other guys, of course, who plunge forward, saying whatever crosses their mind. These guys seem to be incapable of saying anything that doesn't appear gross, and the vocabulary at their disposal seems straight out of a porn flick. What you need to remember before you make any judgments is that they are probably simply inexperienced in having conversations about sex. Sometimes the shyest guy will be the one using the most primitive language.

The most important thing for a woman to remember is that she needs to stay straightforward and direct. Don't be afraid, and just say what's on your mind. Every conversation you have will open the door to future conversations. It's also important for a woman to couch her concerns in a positive way. Don't say, "I really have a serious problem with our sex life," or "I don't like the way you do such and such." Instead say, "There are so many things about our sex life that I love, and I'm so excited by you. In fact, being with you makes me realize how much I like sex. I also think sex could be even better between us, and I've read about these new techniques. I wonder if you are willing to join me in learning some of them together."

I have found for me that it pays to be totally honest, even if it might be awkward. I don't generally go out of my way to stroke anybody's ego, but I think you can usually put a positive spin on things and still maintain your integrity. The point you want to make is this: "I care about our sex life because I care about you. Because I care, I want us to be the best together that we can be."

Many women are afraid that they will sound demanding in bed. I don't think that's a realistic concern. All you have to say is "I'd really like it if you would do that same thing, only just a little slower." Or "You know, I had this fantasy at work today, and in it you were doing (fill in the blank) to me, and I was doing (fill it in). It was just great." You want the following message to get across to the man in your life: "You are the man I want in my bed, and I want us both to be happy and fulfilled."

REALIZE THAT SEX IS NOT A SPECTATOR SPORT

Sex is an athletic activity and, like all athletic activities, it requires certain physical skills and abilities that may not always come naturally. The exercises that follow are ones that you would learn if you were to visit a sex therapist. They are tried and true and I can attest to the fact that they really work. With male clients, I would almost immediately start telling them about the sexual exercises that make a difference. The one piece of advice I always give all women is:

Exercise your sexual muscles and, if it is at all possible, show him how to exercise his.

When I first started to be trained in doing sexual therapy, I was still under the impression that sex was all about hormones, attraction, and lust. It didn't take long for my original teachers to show me that more is required. Good sex is at least partially dependent on knowing what to do and being able to do it.

When I am talking to a man who is having premature ejaculations or a man or a woman who is having weak orgasms, I always tell them about PC exercises. I know the term "PC exercises" doesn't sound very sexy, but trust me, these exercises make all the difference.

This really is the most important sexual exercise.

Both you and your male partner have a pubococcygeal (PC) muscle. The PC muscle is what spasms when you have an orgasm. It does the same thing for your partner when he has an orgasm or ejaculates. These exercises, which help strengthen the PC muscle, are sometimes called Kegels because they were developed by an obstetrician whose last name was Kegel. When I worked with men who wanted to have more control over their erections, one of the first exercises I discussed with them was one that involved the PC muscle. A guy with a well-developed PC muscle can have stronger erections and ejaculations.

For women, a strong PC muscle tightens and tones your vagina; it improves your ability to have orgasm as well as the quality of the ones you have. (Being able to consciously flex your PC muscle at the moment of orgasm intensifies the feeling.) For all women, particularly when they are pregnant or older, these exercises help with bladder control. The other nifty benefit of these exercises is that they help make it possible for you to voluntarily contract and release your vagina during intercourse, a little parlor trick your partner will appreciate. If you are into faking orgasms (although with a strong PC, you shouldn't ever have to do so), being able to create little spasms in your vagina will make it almost impossible for a guy to figure out that you deserve an Academy Award.

If a guy's PC muscle is toned and strong, he will have stronger sensations in the genital area; he will have more control over his erections and be significantly less likely to have premature ejaculation;

he will have better ejaculation control and stronger orgasms; .
works at it, he may also be able to have multiple orgasms. Men wit.
strong PC muscles also have improved prostate health. That's because men who have more complete ejaculations are less likely to
have problems with enlarged prostates as they grow older.

PC muscle exercises for women

1. Locate the PC muscle: Place a finger inside your vagina about
up to the first knuckle. Make believe you are urinating and want to
stop the flow. Feel the muscle that tightens around your finger when
you do this. This is the PC muscle. Once you have located the PC
muscle, you should be able to find it without using your fingers.

2. Flex and relax the PC muscle: Squeeze the PC muscle and
hold it for two seconds. Relax the PC muscle and let it be for two
seconds.

*3. Repeat this process five to twenty-five times and do it three times
a day*: The PC muscle tires easily, so it might be advisable to start
with five to ten reps three times a day. The good news is the PC
muscle tones very quickly so within a few weeks, you should be able
to work your way up to twenty-five reps. Try to keep your breathing
relaxed and even while you are doing these exercises.

The wonderful thing about PC exercises is that you can do them
without anyone realizing that you are doing them. You can do
them at your desk, while you are making dinner, or while you are
driving your car. In short, you can pretty much do them at any time
of day or night.

PC muscle exercises for men

1. Locate the PC muscle: Use two fingers, and gently place
them behind your testicles. Now pretend that you are urinating

the flow. The muscle that you squeeze to do
scle. While you are urinating, practice stopping
flow. Do this several times. Make sure you
re the PC muscle is located and how you can
control it.

2. Flex and release the PC muscle: Squeeze the PC muscle and hold it for two seconds. Relax the PC muscle and let it be for two seconds.

3. Repeat this process five to twenty-five times and do it three times a day: The same thing is true for men as it is with women: The PC muscle tires easily, so it might be advisable to start with five to ten reps three times a day. The good news for most guys is that the PC muscle tones very quickly. Within a few weeks, he should easily be able to do twenty-five reps three times a day.

Guys should be sure that they have isolated the PC muscle and that they are not tightening their abdomens, buttocks, or facial muscles as they exercise. They need to remember to relax and breathe evenly as they squeeze and relax the PC.

When a guy's PC is toned and strong, he should be able to hold back his ejaculation simply by flexing the muscle. The other thing he needs to be aware of is that if he is flexing it involuntarily, he will stop his ejaculation, and he may not understand what is happening.

Talking to men about doing PC exercises

If you would like to talk to a man about doing PC exercises, the first thing you need to do is relax. It's not such a big deal. Men know that women read magazines like *Cosmo*; they know that they read books that give advice like this. All you have to do is tell him that you read about these simple exercises that will make sex better for both of you. Here's a fun way to introduce this conversation:

YOU: Look at my face. Can you tell that I'm exercising muscles in my vagina?

HIM: No . . .

YOU: Well, I am. If you're really good, I'll let you put a finger in my vagina so you can feel what I'm doing.

HIM: What's that?

YOU: Honest! I read this in a book. If I exercise these muscles, I'll have better orgasms. If you exercise your own muscles, you will have more control over those fabulous erections of yours that I love so much. It says that some men even have multiple orgasms. Honest, I swear.

This kind of conversation should get his attention.

Sensate focus: The very best exercise to increase sensuality and sexual awareness

I admit it, I have been extraordinarily successful in helping to turn hundreds of men who had major problems in bed into men who could easily get my good lovemaking seal of approval. Some exercises and techniques absolutely work! This is true when the guy has very specific problems, and it is also true if his biggest issue is that he is either ho-hum or merely clueless. The two most effective exercises you can do with a partner are *sensate focus* and *peaking*.

Sensate focus is a system of exercises and techniques that were originally developed by the famous sex researchers and therapists William Masters and Virginia Johnson. I cannot put enough emphasis on how powerful these exercises can be in improving any couple's sexual relationship.

These exercises were first developed to treat common sexual

…ms such as premature ejaculations, erection difficulties, and …ems with female arousal and orgasm. The goal of sensate focus was to help couples increase their sensuality and awareness of each while removing the burden of performance pressure.

Since the days when Masters and Johnson were doing their groundbreaking work, a great deal has changed about sensate focus. Over the years, my colleagues and I have put together some guidelines and developed many specific exercises to be used for different concerns. Sensate focus refers to a particular way of sensual touching. Sensate focus is very flexible because you can use these guidelines for touching any part of the body. These techniques can also be used during self-touch.

To do a sensate focus exercise, all you and your partner have to do is agree that you will take turns caressing each other's body for a specified period of time following the basic principles of sensate focus.

Here are the basic principles of sensate focus:

1. Touch your partner for your own pleasure: When you touch your partner, do it in a way that feels good to you. Don't worry about what your partner is feeling or thinking. Tell him, "If I do something that bothers you or hurts you, let me know." Otherwise, this is about touching for your own pleasure.

2. Focus on sensation: Whether you are touching your partner's face, his arm, his hand, or his penis, close your eyes and focus all your attention on what your partner's skin feels like. Touching your partner really slowly will help you concentrate. This type of touch is called a caress. Keep in mind that when you touch your partner, you are trying to convey love through your touch.

3. Take the pressure off both of you: Don't look for or expect a particular response either from your partner or yourself. Try to have no expectations about erections, ejaculations, or orgasms. This is about touch.

4. *Stay in the here and now*: Don't think about what happened in the past and don't think about what might be happening in five or ten minutes. Let go of all your thoughts about anything else in the world except what you are doing in the moment. When your mind starts to wander off to other thoughts, bring it back to what you are feeling in the present moment. If you are having difficulty staying focused, slow down. Bring the speed with which you are touching your partner down to half of what it was before.

5. *Remember, this works best if one partner is active while the other remains passive*: This may seem weird and selfish at first, but it takes your sexuality back to its most basic dimensions and helps you pay attention to what you are feeling.

6. *Stay as relaxed as you can*: Relaxation is the key to sensate focus. Remember to take deep calming breaths.

You can use sensate focus touching on any part of your partner's body, and he can use it on any part of yours. All you need to do is find a comfortable body position and stroke any part of your partner's body as slowly as you can, staying focused the whole time. You can touch his face, his back, his front, and his genitals. All that matters is that you are both getting pleasure from what is taking place. Try this a few times and discover why sensate focus is called sensual massage.

Try oral sex using sensate focus techniques.

Here's how you do this: Your partner stays passive. Tell him, "I'm going to give you a massage so you just need to close your eyes, relax, and tell me if I do anything that bothers you." Then slowly caress his penis with your hand with some baby oil. This is a great exercise for any male problems. If you are trying to improve his skills, tell him, "I'm showing you how I like to be touched."

(Keep a warm washcloth handy so you can wipe off the baby oil if you can't stand the taste, or use one of those flavored sexual lubricants that are now available.) Then do oral sex on him for twenty minutes. Stay focused on what you like to do. If he has PE, back off to another part of his body if he becomes too aroused. If he has erection issues, ignore the state of his penis. Give his penis and testicles a caress with your tongue. If you want him to become a better lover, keep teasing his penis until he's about ready to explode.

Combine the magic of peaking with sensate focus.

Peaking is a way of becoming more aware of your own sexual response and patterns as well as those of your partner. In the first chapter, we started talking about stages of arousal. Now we're going to put it into practice.

Think of sexual arousal on a 1 to 10 scale. In this case:

1—represents no arousal

2–3—you are starting to feel intermittent mild twinges of arousal

4–5—arousal is still at a low level, but it is constant

6–7—you are seriously aroused and would have a difficult time stopping

8—very, very aroused with a quickened heartbeat

9—impossible to stop; you are ready to pop

Before you try peaking with a partner, you need to get a better understanding of your own levels of arousal by practicing self-touch with a genital caress. You can use a vibrator or dildo if you want. Go through all the levels of arousal to see what it feels like and also see how long it takes you to get from one stage to the next. You might discover some interesting things about yourself. For example, maybe it takes you a long time to go from 2–4, but once you get to

7, you are on a train and it's not going to stop! This is all good information to know for when you are with a partner.

Time to peak with a partner

Once you have a better sense of your own arousal pattern, it's time to become more familiar with your partner's. Tell your partner about using the 1–10 system of becoming more aware of your arousal. Then ask him if he will agree to do an exercise with you in which you stimulate him manually and orally and he tells you what his arousal level is. Tell him you want to get him excited to a certain arousal level and then back off so his level goes down; then, of course, you will stimulate him some more. All he has to do is assign numbers to his arousal and let you know where he is. Remember that when he gets to a 7 or 8, he is going to be on the way to having an orgasm and will not want to turn back.

Men sometimes start out not expecting to like this exercise. They think it's going to be mechanical, but once they start doing it and discover how sensual and exciting it can be, they usually love it. Peaking is a great exercise for PE, erection problems, and delayed ejaculation. If he indicates that he isn't willing to participate in terms of letting you know his level of arousal, you can still do this on your own. Just tell him to relax and you will give him a massage. You can adjust your touch according to his breathing and heart rate, which you can feel by putting your head on his chest.

The he-can't-help-falling-in-love-with-you sensate focus exercise

Tell your guy that you're going to do a sensual massage on him that will take about an hour. Tell him to lie on his stomach. Start touching his back using sensate focus techniques. Tell him not to move or talk. Make sure the phone and television are off and try not to have any distractions in the room. Caress him lightly and do it so that it pleases you too. Focus completely on how it feels to touch his body. When you turn him over, do the same thing on the front of his body, and slowly begin focusing on his genitals. Use some baby oil on his genitals and do the peaking process, backing off when he gets aroused, and then moving back to his penis again. Climb on top and slowly thrust your way to orgasm. If he wants to move, just tell him this is your thing and he can just relax and enjoy. If he can go all the way to orgasm in this fashion, it will show him a different way of making love. When you are on top of him, gaze into each other's eyes. Warning! This exercise is very powerful, so don't do it with somebody unless you are sure you want to have him fall in love with you.

BE FAMILIAR WITH THE BEST POSITIONS

The basic positions are *male superior* (missionary), *female superior*, *side to side*, and *rear entry*. There are unlimited combinations and variations of these, not to mention the positions you might use if you were having sex in an unusual location—a hot tub, chair, or on top of the kitchen table. There are different motivations for using the different positions. Obviously, you want to use the ones that give you the most physical and psychological arousal. For physical arousal, those would be the male superior and the female superior because they are the most intimate. Many women like the emotional feeling of the man being on top. It depends on your mood and what you are into. There are times, for example, when you might be very turned on by the rear entry position because it's kind of primitive.

When you are with some men in bed, the position you use may

not always be your choice. You may prefer to use a certain position based on sexual issues, physical limitations, or penis and body size.

The best position with a man who . . .

. . . is much taller or heavier than you is **female superior**.

. . . has a small penis is **butterfly** (see below) or **side to side** because your pelvises are closer this way. Also, with the butterfly position, your vagina is somewhat shortened.

. . . has a large penis is **female superior**, so you have control of how fast it goes in and how much it goes in. The straight missionary position will sometimes also work because the woman's legs are flat and the vagina is elongated in this position.

. . . has PE is **side to side** because it is the least arousing.

. . . has erection issues is **butterfly** (see below) because it is easiest to enter with a less-than-hard penis or **side to side** because your pelvises are close so there is less possibility of fallout.

. . . has delayed ejaculations is **butterfly** because it is arousing or **rear entry** because it's the easiest to thrust hard and get a lot of friction.

. . . has cardiac issues or has just had surgery is the **female superior** position.

. . . has arthritis or orthopedic problems is **side to side** because neither person has to support their own weight.

Learn the butterfly position (my favorite)

I sometimes call this the "vase" position. That's because of the joke about the beautiful woman whose boyfriend sends her an extravagant bouquet of flowers, which are delivered to her office. One of her co-workers sees the flowers and says, "If my boyfriend sent me flowers like that, you can be sure I'd be spending the next week on my back with my knees behind my shoulders!" The woman who received the flowers replies, "Why, don't you have a vase?"

The butterfly position is a variation of the man-on-top missionary position, but that doesn't mean that it's boring or old hat. In fact, it's my favorite position because it delivers great orgasms.

For this position, the woman lies on her back, tilts her pelvis and puts her legs as far back as she can without becoming uncomfortable. If she is very flexible, she can bend her knees so that they are almost up to her shoulders. This allows her vagina to be open wide. The farther up she gets her knees, the better, because at this angle, her vagina points almost straight up. If the woman wants to put a pillow under her hips, it can help.

The man kneels between her legs so that he doesn't have to support his weight with his arms and inserts his penis.

I really like this position for the following reasons:

This position causes the vagina to curve. Because of this, the man's penis is able to penetrate deeper and can better stimulate the vagina. If a woman wants a vaginal or uterine orgasm, this is the most likely position for it to happen.

This position gives the man greater control. He can use his penis to switch back and forth between internal strokes and stimulating his partner's clitoris. The man can also use his penis to tease the woman's PC muscle.

Because he isn't using his arms or hands to support his weight, the man can use his hands to alternate between intercourse and masturbation, which is very effective if the man is having a difficult time maintaining an erection or being able to ejaculate.

This position allows for intimate eye contact and when the man leans forward, the couple can kiss.

Both partners can see each other, and both partners can also see the penis going in and out of the vagina, which most men (and many women) find very stimulating.

SOME FINAL WORDS OF ADVICE

Always have a fall-back for when the hormones go south.

Hot, steamy, hot, hot (did I say hot?) sex is great. I love sexual relationships when they are new and so hot that even when you are in a great restaurant, you can't wait to finish dinner before racing home with your hands all over each other and throwing your clothes all over the place as you dive into each other. Enjoy this as long as it lasts! Realize, however, that this kind of sex doesn't last forever. When the hormones and the hunger subside, it's good to have something else up your sleeve. This is when you need a good sensual base to the relationship. I always advise clients to include some sensuality in their sexual encounters even when they are brand new and surging along without any help. Get into the habit of including things like foot massage, back massage, bubble baths, and body oils into your lovemaking from the very beginning. It will improve the quality of your sexual relationship and heighten intimacy. Practices like this also increase trust and openness between romantic partners. All of this allows sex to become a deeper and more connected experience even after the initial hormonal surge starts to disappear.

Remember, you can train a good guy to be a good lover.

But you can't train a creep to be a good guy. I've met a fair number of men who were divine in bed and real creeps in every other area of their lives. These are the guys who are rude to waiters, mean to their children, and vile to their wives, but get them in bed and they become sensual pussycats. Go figure! My often-repeated point is that you can train a good guy to be good in bed, but you can't train a guy who's good in bed to be a good person in other areas.

The bottom line: If you meet a guy who is a good human being with a good personality, and all he has are some sexual problems, don't give up on him. The major lesson I've learned from doing surrogate work and sexual therapy is that sex problems can be cured. Personality problems, on the other hand, are for life.

The key factors are motivation and commitment.

The most sexually clueless guy in the world can become a fabulous lover if he is motivated to change. Nonetheless, I think it's essential for a woman to understand that it might not be a good idea to try to become some kind of sexual saint helping a guy work on his issues unless he is equally committed to the relationship. If he evolves into a fabulous lover and then moves on, you might be a little perturbed. So unless you are okay with this kind of outcome, make sure you are both on the same relationship page, and you are working on the sexual issues together.

Most of the time, his sexual issues are not about you.

I feel fairly safe in assuring you that if he is having sexual difficulties in bed, it's not about you or anything you are doing. Every man has his own set of sexual baggage that he carries with him. He has a very specific medical history and a very specific emotional history. He also has well-established behavior patterns. Unless you met as toddlers in the sandbox, these were in place before you entered his life. If a guy ejaculates too quickly (or not quickly enough) with you, it's highly unlikely he will be any different with any other woman. The same thing is true if he has difficulties with his erection. This is all about him, not about you.

Sometimes it is about you and your attitude.

Your attitude, self-esteem, and confidence can make any sexual encounter great. If I like a man enough to be in bed with him, I always assume it's going to be positive, good, and possibly even great. And if it's not, in the larger scheme of things, what's the big deal? You can learn something from every sexual experience you have, even if it's not so great. Sometimes you learn something about men; sometimes you learn something about sex; sometimes you learn something about yourself. Just remember to stay positive and confident.

Be honest about what you want and don't want.

Don't change your personality because you think the guy in your bed will like you better if you do. Don't change your likes or dislikes for every guy you want to be with. Otherwise you will find yourself living a lie in a relationship that isn't really satisfying you. Most men are prepared to compromise to please a woman they like, but let them know. It's very difficult to tell somebody six months or a year down the road, "You know I don't really like that." True intimacy is dependent on honesty.

Don't do anything you really don't want to do.

If you are in a relationship, yes, that calls for a certain amount of compromise on your part. But if you feel that you are being forced to do things in bed that you really hate, don't do it. Never do anything that feels abusive. It's not good for you, and it's not good for the relationship. It goes without saying that you shouldn't do anything that feels hurtful. If a guy slaps you around or is otherwise abusive, run! Do not be a victim and don't set yourself up to be a victim.

Be honest with yourself.

If all you are looking for is a short-term sexual encounter, accept that. If you're really looking for the long-term, big love, don't settle for short-term sex. If you do, there is a good possibility that you will end up feeling horrible about yourself. Go with your gut feeling. You can tell when the relationship feels as though it is intimate and when it is not. If you are looking for intimacy, it's probably best to hold off on sex when you meet a new man (something I have never been able to do), but I still think it's good advice.

If he doesn't want to change, you're not going to make it happen.

Every sex therapist knows that there are some problems with men that you can't solve or change, no matter how hard you try. Sexual compulsions, for example, rarely go away. If you meet a guy with a long-standing fetish/paraphilia, even if he is the sweetest guy in the world, know up front that the chances that he will lose his paraphilia are very slim. The same thing is true if you fall for a man who is really closed off emotionally and is wedded to his sexual patterns, whatever they might be. It is unlikely that you can do anything to change him.

Know that all men are different.

Pick up any one of a dozen popular magazines and you will find articles with titles like "Ten Things *He* Never Wants You to Do in Bed" or "Ten Things *He* Always Wants You to Do in Bed" or even "What *He* Really Wants for Christmas This Year." Read these articles and you'll come away with the impression that all guys are alike, and there is one universal *He*. Yes, I could probably say something along the lines of "All Guys Like Sex," and I would probably be right almost all of the time, but the fact is that if you become sexually involved with enough men, you are going to find one who dreams of celibacy. You simply cannot make generalities or assumptions about men. It's like fingerprints or DNA. Each man is distinctive and different. No two men are going to have the same level of desire; no two men are going to be exactly alike in how they make love; no two men are going to want to do exactly the same thing in exactly the same way. To complicate matters even further, the same man is going to be different at different stages of his life. The shy, never-been-kissed nineteen-year-old guy can evolve into a thirty-year-old who has sex with a different woman every night, and the twenty-five-year-old stud can turn into the forty-year-old with low sexual desire.

Don't judge a book by its cover.

One important piece of advice I would give all women: You can't tell what a man will be like in bed (or for that matter anywhere else) based upon how he looks or how he acts when you first meet him. The great-looking guy who is fearless about making sexy conversation could turn out to really lack sizzle in the sack. So could the guy wearing the Rolex and the world's most perfectly pressed clothes. On the other hand, I've been with some men who looked completely ordinary and unassuming, and they turned out to be fabulous, confident lovers who really knew what to do on a mattress, be it a king-size pillow top or a twin-size rollaway.

Remember, he's only human.

It doesn't matter whether he is completely lovable or totally infuriating, the world's best lover or among the world's worst, the common denominator between the guy in your bed and all the other guys in the world is that they are all human. I realize that you may be looking at that sentence right now and thinking, "Duh, so what else is new?" But think about it for a minute: As women, don't we sometimes give men more power in our lives than they really have? Don't we sometimes think about them as though they are larger than life or as though they belong to a different species?

Yes, the man in your life may be able to do things that make you feel happy and fulfilled, and yes, he may also be able to do things that make you feel miserable and out of control. Yes, he may have an uncanny instinct about which of your erogenous zone buttons to push to bring your body to life, and yes, he may also have an unerring instinct about missing the buttons you want pushed. Yes, he is important to you, but no matter how high he ranks in your personal world, it still does not give him superhuman powers. The typical guy is just as confused about his sexuality and how to put it together as you are. You may be thinking of him as a larger-than-life superhero who knows what he is doing, while he may be regarding himself as a vulnerable naked guy, stripped of his cape, working his way through a maze of kryptonite. When you and the man in your bed are not making beautiful music together, remember, he's only human and you're only human, but together you should be able to find a human solution to any sexual difficulties you are experiencing as a couple.